Lavender Hair

VICTORIA JACKSON

Lavender

Hair

❧ 21 ☙

DEVOTIONS FOR
WOMEN WITH
BREAST CANCER

BroadStreet
P U B L I S H I N G

BroadStreet Publishing® Group, LLC
Racine, Wisconsin, USA
BroadStreetPublishing.com

Lavender Hair: 21 Devotions for Women with Breast Cancer

ISBN-13: 978-1-4245-5562-8 (softcover)
ISBN-13: 978-1-4245-5563-5 (e-book)

Stock or custom editions of BroadStreet Publishing titles may be purchased in bulk for educational, business, ministry, fundraising, or sales promotional use. For information, please e-mail info@broadstreetpublishing.com.

Cover design by Chris Garborg at garborgdesign.com
Cover photo by Brandon Wood at indiebling.com
Typesetting by Katherine Lloyd at theDESKonline.com

Printed in the United States of America

17 18 19 20 21 5 4 3 2 1

contents

WHO, ME?

"For with God nothing shall be impossible."

LUKE 1:37

*W*ho me? I can't write a "devotional." I'm too bitter and jaded and sarcastic ... and skeptical.

But, every time a bitter, jaded, sarcastic, or skeptical thought comes into my head, a Bible verse flies in and kicks it out. *Shoo!*

Is that what a "devotional" is? A personal story where the Word of God saves the day?

Yes?

Well, I can do that!

God's Word has been the light of my path my whole life. Sometimes, at the fork in the road, I've taken the wrong path, but His hand has guided me back to Him and to the narrow way.

Sometimes when I've taken a stand for Christ, I've lost career opportunities and friends. And my thoughts become, *Maybe they're right. I am nuts! I believe in a fairy tale! God is invisible!* But then, I stumble upon the blue robin's eggs in a nest in the evergreen tree in my backyard and I realize I am in awe of this Great Designer. I watch my grandchildren laugh and play and I think about their mother's little heartbeat that started in my stomach. I watch the archaeologists in the Middle East uncovering Sodom and Gomorrah. I hear scientists trying to explain DNA. I study the Bible and am amazed at the new things I'm discovering after all these years. "I know whom I have believed" (2 Timothy 1:12), and I know He will finish the good work He started in me (Philippians 1:6).

Then, I doubt again the next day.

I mean, the wooden sign that sits under my TV in my bedroom, the sign I look at every night says, *"I believe. Help my unbelief." Mark 9:24. Boom!* A Bible verse kicked the doubt right out of my head, again. So, I guess I can write a devotional. I have felt the presence of God.

Ever since I was six years old and realized that the preacher at Carol City Baptist Church wasn't just talking to the congregation— God was talking to me personally, and "God so loved the world" (John 3:16) meant "God loved Vicki"—I have gone to the Word of God for the answers to all my questions. "As for God, his way is perfect: The Lord's Word is flawless; He shields all who take refuge in Him" (Psalm 18:30).

When I got cancer last year, my Bible training came in very handy. I needed it. And, I had to live the Word, not just read it, memorize it, or talk about it.

This is my testimony. I pray that "the God of hope [will] fill you with all joy and peace as you trust in him, so that you may overflow with hope by the power of the Holy Spirit" (Romans 15:13).

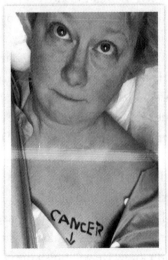

Double mastectomy day, Nov. 17, 2015.

COUGHING AT ZANIES

> I can do all things through Christ who strengthens me.
>
> PHILIPPIANS 4:13 ESV

I can't stop coughing. I'm lying on the couch in the green room at Zanie's Comedy Club in Nashville. It's October 8, 2015. In just a few moments, I have to perform a forty-five-minute comedy routine in front of a live audience. But I can barely say one sentence without coughing! I'm drinking tea with lemon and honey, sucking on cough drops, and praying, then repeating the cycle.

I'm trying out some new jokes:

For some reason, a lot of people think I'm political! What happened is, I went to the town hall to renew my tags, and I got in the wrong line. They wanted twenty-five signatures. I said, "To drive?" Then, they asked me which political party I was in. I don't know why they call it a party. Everyone is fighting all the time. I picked Tea Party, because it sounded the most fun. They said, "Who are you voting for?" I said, "Earl Grey." I thought it was about the tea!

Stand-up comedy is the scariest thing I've ever done. No, auditioning for *Saturday Night Live* (SNL) was. No, doing a back handspring on the four-inch-wide balance beam when I was twelve years old. No, getting held up by a robber with a gun in a parking lot in downtown Los Angeles in 1980. No, being told I had cancer. No … uh, marriage is the hardest!

3

You know, when you get cancer, it doesn't make all of your other ongoing problems go away. It just shuffles around your "trials and tribulations" list, and cancer jumps up on top.

And cancer can make your current list of challenges harder or easier. Some problems fade under the magnitude of the word *fatal*. Other problems are exacerbated. My oncologist said weak marriages don't survive breast cancer. Of my four married cancer friends, two of the four marriages did not survive. My marriage is a daily spiritual battle. We pray through each day. So far, we are still married. Twenty-five years. One day at a time.

Just keepin' it real.

I'm staring at a picture of Bob Dylan on the green room wall. The "green room" is where entertainers wait before they go onstage. Green is considered the calming color. This green room is beige. Someone pops their head in and says, "Five minutes."

Cough, cough. "Thank you," I say. *Cough, cough.*

I wonder if Bob Dylan ever went onstage with a cough.

The enemy has tried everything to take me down, so cancer doesn't surprise me. He tried temptation, ambition, addiction, discouragement, betrayal, divorce, peer pressure, loneliness, and even success—anything to take my eyes off of Jesus. Ephesians 6:12 says, "For we do not wrestle against flesh and blood, but against principalities, against powers, against the rulers of the darkness of this age, against spiritual hosts of wickedness in the heavenly places" (ESV).

My dad was a PE teacher and a gymnastics coach and he taught me to be brave at a very young age. Our backyard was full of little girls doing flips on our trampoline, bars, and beam—the gym in our backyard. I cracked my vertebrae once, knocked my breath out falling off the high bar, broke a finger, and had knee pain caused by Osgood-Schlatter disease.

I never questioned doing dangerous "tricks." It was the family business. My dad would spot me. I trusted him. I competed in meets. My palms were sweaty. My stomach full of butterflies. Dad always said, "It doesn't matter if you win or lose, it's whether you do your best. If you do your best, you're a winner."

So, Dad taught me to be brave mentally and physically. But, also spiritually. I was taught to witness to people, to tell the lost about Jesus. At Dade Christian School I was graded on my perfect memorization of Bible verses, the King James version, with all the beautiful thees and thous; so for the rest of my life, these Bible verses pop into my head, and always at the perfect moment. Especially, when I'm scared.

In my childhood red leather Bible are scribbled notes and dates of the worries I was giving to God. The worries changed as I grew older. It's fun to go back and look at them and see how God answered my prayers. He gave me victory every time. And, He always will.

Going onstage is stressful. With a cough, it's even more stressful. People paid money, they got babysitters, and they're all sitting there waiting. The show must go on. There's a rhythm to a "set." I'll try not to cough on the punch lines.

I hear my name announced, and I walk into the spotlight. *Cough, cough.*

The enemy, who comes to steal, to kill, and to destroy (John 10:10), keeps trying to take me out one way or another, because he knows I love Jesus.

But thanks be to God! He gives us the victory through our Lord Jesus Christ. (1 Corinthians 15:57)

TIP: Play the song "Victor's Crown" by Darlene Zschech on a loop and sing loudly while wearing a knight-in-armor costume and looking in the mirror. Prepare for battle.

RED FLAG: UH OH

"Be not afraid, neither be thou dismayed for
the Lord thy God is with thee whithersoever thou goest."

JOSHUA 1:9 KJV

*C*oughing in my car on the way home from Zanies, I thought about Jim McCawley, the talent scout for *The Tonight Show Starring Johnny Carson* who "discovered" me at the Variety Arts Center in 1983 where I was doing stand-up. He gave me my big break. He preinterviewed me twenty times before my twenty appearances on the show. In 1992, while having me guest star on the short-lived *Vicki!* show with Vicki Lawrence, he showed me a big scar down his chest and, with a quizzical smile and wide eyes, told me he had just had a grapefruit-sized tumor removed from his lungs. Cancer. He wasn't a smoker but had spent years of long nights in smoky comedy clubs discovering talent for Johnny Carson. Jim McCawley died of lung cancer at age fifty-four.

I had spent many nights in those same comedy clubs working on my set and breathing second-hand smoke.

Uh oh.

Physical and emotional pain are knit together. The constant coughing and my thoughts of Jim were giving way to fear. "Thou wilt keep him in perfect peace, whose mind is stayed on thee" (Isaiah 26:3 KJV) was the verse that popped into my mind and kicked out those thoughts of fear that boiled and bubbled there.

During my set at Zanies, Husband (that's what I'll call him) had refused to play the piano for me. He doesn't support my show biz passions. It's a constant frustration to me. I love the stage. He hates it.

Whenever my marriage gets too difficult, I make up jokes about it. Husband helps me write the jokes. One of the best remedies for our disagreements, since we are opposites in every way, is laughter.

At Zanies that night I had tried out a few new ones:

Husband isn't good onstage. He only has one facial expression. Cop face. He's a cop. Good for arresting people. And, he's Chickasaw. Totem Pole. The house is on fire! Deadpan. We won the lottery! Same face. Good for a cop, not for show business. I told Husband that. He said, "I don't want to be in show business!" We've been working on Husband's expressions. He has five now: (1) his default face (scary, deadpan), (2) toothy smile, (3) tiny smile, (4) surprise, and (5) Blue Steel from the Ben Stiller movie Zoolander.

We've had seven marriage therapists. They all committed suicide. Actually, one exploded, so it's only six suicides. I'm starting to feel like a serial killer.

Husband can't leave his police personality at work. Sometimes in bed he puts his arm around me and says, "Do you have any idea why I pulled you over?" Once, I overslept, and he drew a chalk outline around me.

When I'm having husband problems and feeling alone, I remember Isaiah 54:5–6 (NASB):

For your husband is your Maker,
Whose name is the LORD of hosts;
And your Redeemer is the Holy One of Israel,
Who is called the God of all the earth.
For the LORD has called you,
Like a wife forsaken and grieved in spirit,
Even like a wife of one's youth when she is rejected.

See, God knows what I'm feeling. And, He loves me.

God is my God, not Husband. God will be my support when all others have failed me. I am to respect and honor Husband, but worship God. I am learning to care about God's opinion of me more than Husband's opinion. Usually, if I'm pleasing God, I am simultaneously pleasing Husband, but not always. In "This Journey Is My Own" Sara Groves sings about living and breathing as if God alone were in the audience. During marital gridlock, I've learned to first get my priorities straight with God, and then I can carry on with the daily wifely requirements of selflessness and forgiveness toward Husband.

I somehow made it through the Zanies hour of talking.

The next day at the gym, I was still coughing and the other people on the elliptical machines kept moving away from me. Sigh. Better do something. I never went to the doctor for checkups. I don't have a primary doctor. I don't trust them—they make too many mistakes. They are "practicing" medicine. But, three days earlier, I had felt a little numb spot near my left underarm area. That was weird. I even mentioned it to Husband.

I guess the strange numb spot added to the cough compelled me to the nearest walk-in clinic. I was sweaty from the gym, which I know is rude, but I thought I would chicken out if I didn't go see a doctor right then. It was midday in a work week. I figured everyone would be at work, so hardly anyone to notice my sweaty self.

I knew if I went home to shower first I might get distracted with:

- *YouTube surfing.* I want to learn more about everything, so I spend hours researching such topics as the Illuminati, singers, atheists, art, Édith Piaf, eschatology, Paris, castles, the Dead Sea Scrolls, celebrity gossip, CERN, and the mysterious Bob Dylan.
- *Garage shifting.* I shift my junk from one side of the garage to the other side and think I've organized it.

- *Housekeeping.* I start to clean out a drawer, get distracted by *FOX News*, get my curiosity sparked, and start to research why world leaders have recently visited the Antarctica, which leads me to realize I've forgotten my password again. This starts the …
- *Password reset phase.* Hours can be consumed in this phase. I write my new passwords down, lose the paper, punch them into my cell phone, drop my cell into the toilet, and repeat the cycle.

Five years before, around menopause, my breasts had suddenly started growing, and the left one had developed a weird dent in it. I figured it was just misshapen fat or a slipped implant. I got busy and forgot about it. It couldn't be cancer. I wasn't sick. I didn't need a doctor to tell me that cancer didn't run in our family and there was no lump, just a dent.

But now was different. I think there was a small inner voice telling me something serious was wrong inside my body. I didn't know what. I just knew now was the time to do something. And I knew God would be with me no matter the outcome.

Be anxious for nothing, but in everything by prayer and supplication with thanksgiving let your requests be made known to God. And the peace of God, which surpasses all comprehension, will guard your hearts and your minds in Christ Jesus. (Philippians 4:6–7 NASB)

TIP: Get regular doctor checkups. Bonus points for taking a shower before you go. And, don't go to the gym if you're coughing on everybody. My bad. My bad. My bad.

WAITING ROOM:
I'M JUST A STATISTIC

Why are you cast down, O my soul?
And why are you disquieted within me?
Hope in God;
For I shall yet praise Him,
The help of my countenance and my God.

PSALM 43:5 KJV

I am whisked into the inner sanctum of the walk-in clinic, and I apologize about my gym clothes. I tell the male nurse about my cough. He starts scribbling something, and then I casually mention, "I have this numb spot near my underarm. I don't know if it's related. Maybe it's my twenty-five-year-old silicone breast implant leaking or a lymph gland fighting this cough? Might as well ask since I'm here."

The male nurse touches the spot and says, "You have to go to the breast clinic immediately."

"You feel a lump? I don't feel a lump."

He looks serious, hands me a paper, and says, "This is where my wife goes."

Goes?

I'm sitting in the lobby at the Vanderbilt Breast Clinic waiting to be examined for a second time. Didn't look good the first time. I glance around. There are two old men waiting for their wives and many husband-less middle-aged women who look just like me. Lumpy. A bit worn out. Serious-faced. This isn't an Auburn University theatre major party. *Hmph.* I have tried very hard to be healthy (gymnastics and salad), to be special, have a fun life, or a bedazzled one. But, I'm just a statistic. I'm a big old fat cliché.

I try to be nonchalant. But death is looming. I can feel it.

God will know how to shake off this icky feeling. I ask God to speak to me as I shuffle through my Bible. This verse pops out: "Hope in God" (Psalm 43:5). It spins into a ukulele ditty. And, my heart feels happy.

My name is called, and I bounce into the private inner lobby. I'm told to undress and put on a beige robe that is identical to the other fifteen middle-aged women who are flipping through magazines, awaiting their MRI, pretending not to be there. They are not looking at their magazines or to the left or the right. They are in their own internal, personal cells. The intense focus of staving off fear permeates the room. No one makes eye contact, speaks, or acknowledges each other.

I do not like this moment. It is so icky that it's almost funny. It looks like the set of an *SNL* comedy sketch. I expect something funny to happen, because the setup is so serious. I feel fear too, but strangely, I also feel happy inside. Hope in God. I am on an adventure with God. I don't know what this journey will look like, but I know the end is swell. I'll be with Him. And, He owns the universe. I'm writing a song about Him in my head. I love when that happens.

"For me to live is Christ, and to die is gain" (Philippians 1:21 ESV) pops into my mind. I have heard, read, written, memorized, spoken, and sung that verse all my life. Now, I am living it.

I think of the apostle Paul in prison awaiting his martyrdom and other Christians who face death for the cause of Christ. I am not doing that. I am just facing death because of bad luck, bad lifestyle choices, or genetics. Nothing to brag about. But the same kind of impending doom.

Every time fear creeps into my mind, that verse, Philippians 1:21, flies in and kicks it out! *Shoo!*

My name is called, and I'm told to lie down and open my robe.

The MRI nurse looks very serious when I look at the black spiderlike blob on the screen and say, "Is that what cancer looks like?"

She cautiously replies, "It can."

I do not want this. This is not good. Unpleasant. Gloomy. Bad. Darkness is pressing down on me.

I try to think of hope. Only thing I can come up with is—Jesus. Will I trust Him even if I have cancer? Even if He doesn't heal me?

My friend Lisa once said to me, "Trusting God, really trusting God, believing that He means the best for you and that He has your back, when you're holding the hand of your twenty-year-old sister who is dying of breast cancer, that's trusting God."

Putting my clothes back on, I think about how funny it is that the Vanderbilt Breast Clinic is located inside a mall and next to a movie theater, like it's just another fun stop in the day of a blessed American—pedicure, movie, new dress, ice cream cone, cancer treatment, Manolo Blahnik shoes …

On the way to my car, I see a wonderful leopard bath robe in the window of TJ Maxx. I am a patient now. I have to have it!

I am still hopeful that it's just a small thing that can easily be cut out and forgotten. But a dark cloud is forming over me.

I will soon find out I have stage 3C breast cancer that has been growing inside me for five to ten years and that got aggressive when it moved to my lymph nodes. All twenty-six nodes were removed from my left side when they found nine of them had cancer. This leaves me with a 40 percent chance of getting lymphedema (painful swelling) for life in the left arm.

Sara Groves sings about death in her song "What Do I Know." She says she doesn't know much about heaven, but she knows that to absent from the body is to be present with the Lord (2 Corinthians 5:8). And from what she knows of Him, it must be very good!

TIP: Early detection is the best cure. One out of eight women get breast cancer. I had seven friends who didn't have breast cancer. Uh oh. And, most breast cancer patients have no genetic link.

DIaGnOSIS
WITH a SOUTHern DrawL

And we know that all things work together
for good to them that love God, to them who
are the called according to his purpose.

ROMANS 8:28 KJV

*I*n the movies, people find out they have cancer at a big desk, sitting
near a loved one, across from a doctor who looks very serious.
Then they start to cry. The way I found out I had cancer was a swirly,
gradual, round-about kind of way, in stages.

Like how hors d'oeuvres whet your appetite and slowly start up
your tummy, getting it ready for a nice big serious meal. Cancer was
partially announced to me on the phone by a slow-drawling Southern
belle named Tracey, who used big words and made it sound so sweet
and delicious that when I hung up, I was as happy as if I'd just won a
free pecan pie at the county fair.

"Your biopsy results show a slow-growing, most common ductal
[*something, something*] malignant ..."

That's the bad thing, right?

"No proof that it's traveled, so it probably won't need chemo, but
might ..."

Sounded okay. I'm an optimist.

Everyone over forty has that deep fear in the back of their head—
cancer. Every time you sip a Diet Coke with all those chemicals in it, the
chemicals you can use to clean ship decks—cancer. Every time you eat

a GMO (genetically modified organism), or chicken from a fast food drive-through, knowing the chicken was kept in a dark little jail and fed hormones to fatten him up—cancer. Every time you read articles that say alcohol or luncheon meats or sugar causes cancer, you wince and cross your fingers behind your back as you sneak a puff from someone's Marlboro Ultra Light or lick that Orange Cream See's Lollypop—cancer. Then you find out your one healthy habit, unsalted sunflower seeds, contain phytoestrogen and estrogen feeds breast cancer.

So you throw your hands up and just quit trying to not "catch" cancer.

Before age forty, you're indestructible.

"We won't really know if the cancer has spread to your lymph nodes until we open you up," says Tracy the Southern Belle.

Open me up? They are going to cut me open. I had been wanting to lose those implants for years but not exactly like this.

The surgery to remove the spiderlike clump was scheduled for as soon as possible. Of course, we had to go through health insurance red tape. I found myself on the phone with a stranger, telling her that cancer was eating me alive, and if she would please just push the paperwork through a little faster, I would really appreciate it and might not literally die. This year.

"There are a lot of people ahead of you in line with the same problems, honey." *Gum smack. Gum smack.*

I was hoping my life was more meaningful than that. Standing in a line.

I knew God must have an important reason for me getting this dire diagnosis. My first thought was: *God must want me to witness to someone in this medical maze.* So, I ordered some leather devotionals, *Daily Light* by Anne Graham Lotz, and gave them to some of the staff at the Vanderbilt Breast Clinic. I had their names engraved on the cover. I know God will use my situation for His glory and for my benefit.

At church, when Balcony Mike (the balcony usher) found out I had cancer, he forced me to meet the worship leader, Debi Selby, because she had just gone through breast cancer. Mike literally pushed me into her, because I was too shy.

I had watched her singing onstage every Sunday, going bald, wearing head scarves, being prayed over, and being healed. I had prayed for her healing, not knowing I was next. Debi hugged me tight and instantly became my cheerleader. She ended up walking through it with me, sending me encouraging texts with Scripture, and giving me her scarves. She even bought me a leopard one. Don't you know all women over fifty love animal prints!

"Chemo? *Pfft!*" she said. "Watch old movies, eat ice cream in bed, spoil yourself." She even brought me homemade split pea soup.

Other friends sent flowers, cards, Bible verses, a patchwork quilt, knitted shawls, and hats. Every gesture of love touched me deeply and stays with me now. Never one to accept help or pity, it was uncomfortable, but I took all the gifts, prayers, and love and was grateful.

At Vanderbilt, a beautiful name for a hospital—sounds like a castle—I am knocked out, so they can put a port in my chest. A box with a pin cushion to receive needles and a tube. This is to keep the veins in my arms from collapsing from overpokage. It is a nuisance, because that is the spot where my granddaughter Dewy lays her head.

A tube comes out of the port and is sewn into an artery in my neck. You can't make this stuff up. I see the little tube under my skin. I'm afraid it will come undone, and blood will squirt everywhere inside me, and I'll drop dead in public somewhere. But, this doesn't happen. It just sits there for a few months, before they surgically remove it.

I feel like a science experiment. I marvel at the advances medicine has made and at the efficiency of the medical staff. They are also kind and professional. They act like they have done this before. I guess I'm not the only person going through this.

I've been trying to have a good attitude about my sudden cancer diagnosis, but, it can be a drag. Friends are finding out and are shocked but not as shocked as me. I feel great physically. I don't have pain or symptoms. Sometimes I wonder if the doctors just made up the whole thing, like a big trick. A conspiracy! How can I have a disease if I feel great? Right?

I think of Tom Hanks' wife, Rita, who was just diagnosed with breast cancer, had surgery, and returned to Broadway, and Olivia Newton John, a twenty-five-year breast cancer survivor. Joan Lunden and Shannon Dougherty were on the cover of *People*, bald. Hey! Why aren't I on the cover of *People*? I'm bald!

It tests your faith in God.

Husband and I discuss the near future. They are going to cut my breasts off. To be honest, they weren't that great. I don't think either one of us will miss them! Well, yeah, we will.

Do we plan a funeral now? Do we fly to Paris? Check items off my bucket list? We've never had this experience before. It's a strange new land. Am I ugly? Is Husband leaving me?

We cannot carry this load. It's too heavy. We pray. We are apprehensive but also have an overwhelming supernatural peace that can only be from Christ.

I look at Husband. Eye to eye. Soul to soul.

Husband says, "One day at a time."

Jesus says, "Do not worry about tomorrow, for tomorrow will worry about itself. Each day has enough trouble of its own." (Matthew 6:34)

TIP: Bring your Bible everywhere. Better yet, put it into your head. Memorize it. It has a happy ending.

maureen and julia

> "Blessed is the man who trusts in the LORD,
> and whose hope is the LORD. For he shall be like a tree
> planted by the waters, which spreads out its roots by the river,
> and will not fear when heat comes; but its leaf will be green,
> and will not be anxious in the year of drought,
> nor will cease from yielding fruit."
>
> JEREMIAH 17:7–8 NKJV

*I*t's interesting to watch people's reaction to my diagnosis. One lady responded, "Does it run in your family?"

"No!"

"Oh no!" she said. "*I* could get it too!"

Twenty years ago, when I found out that Maureen was dying of cancer, my first thought was, *Oh no! I love her!* My second thought was, *Oh no! I could get it! Is God warning me? Is this a foreshadowing of my demise?* Maureen was a fellow gymnast who died at age thirty-six from breast cancer.

I don't know if she drank or smoked. My parents always told me not to drink or smoke. Drinking and smoking—they go together—always made me feel guilty because (1) I am a Christian, and they are considered worldly habits that carnal, immoral people do, and (2) they can cause cancer and our bodies are the temple of God and should be treated that way.

The *Crazy, Sexy Cancer* health guru Kris Carr said in an interview that when she was diagnosed at age thirty-one with inoperable lung and liver cancer, she immediately changed her lifestyle, diet, and thoughts. So did I. I watched her interviews to see if she drank or smoked or did drugs. She said she wouldn't consider herself a "smoker" because she never bought a pack, but there was often one in her hand, and that she wasn't a full-blown "alcoholic" but there were unhealthy substances in her body weekly and her diet was not based on nutrition but on limiting calories. Me too! Many of us spend our youth trying to be skinny, not trying to be healthy.

From her interviews, it sounds like Kris Carr is trusting in herself for her healing and her eternal destiny. I pray she sees Jesus is the way, the truth, and the life. Self as God is a false teaching based on the lie that began in the garden of Eden. "'You won't die!' the serpent replied to the woman. 'God knows that your eyes will be opened as soon as you eat it, and you will be like God'" (Genesis 3:4–5 NLT).

The Bible says to treat my body as the temple of God. I did, until my puberty problems kicked in, and the eating disorders disassembled all sanity and reason and replaced my righteous thinking with lies from the enemy. Lies like "Being skinny is more important than being healthy," "You'll never find a husband or have a show biz career if you aren't thin," and "Eating less and exercising more isn't enough—you need shortcuts, tricks."

Maureen was one of the girls on my dad's team, Jim Jackson's Jumping Jacks Gymnastic Team. Dad, the ex-vaudevillian, trampolinist, juggler, Baptist deacon, PE teacher, and gym coach, took Jesus out of the church and gymnastics out of the gym.

Dad did handstands on the top of his car.

And talked about Jesus while leaning on a gymnastic apparatus.

One day, Dad called me over to the balance beam and asked me to recite John 3:16 to Maureen. I did. I felt a little embarrassed to be reciting the Bible in public but also felt filled with the power of the Holy Spirit. Like we three were on a higher plane, a spiritual plane, as the shallow, insignificant physical world tumbled about us. I think Dad's motives were twofold: he was teaching me how to witness, but he also had a bad memory. We were sweaty and wearing leotards. Maureen was Catholic. She said she'd never heard that Bible verse before. I was proud of my dad for caring about Maureen's soul.

Twenty years later, Maureen appeared at a comedy club where I was doing stand-up. She had a wig and a hat on. She took me in a back room, removed her wig and hat, showed me her bald head, and said, "I have cancer" as if she was still in shock. She wanted my dad's phone number to tell him he was the first person who ever told her about Jesus and that she had just asked Jesus into her heart. The breast cancer went to her brain. She died a year later.

During that year, I sent her letters with encouraging Bible verses:

- "The Lord Jesus will transform our lowly body that it may be conformed to His glorious body" (Philippians 3:20–21 NKJV).
- "Beloved, now are we the sons of God, and it doth not yet appear what we shall be: but we know that, when he shall appear, we shall be like him; for we shall see him as he is" (1 John 3:2 KJV).
- "Jesus said to her, 'I am the resurrection and the life. He who believes in Me, though he may die, he shall live'" (John 11:25 NKJV).

Going through my piles that I shift from one side of my garage to the other, I stumbled upon this e-mail from Maureen's loving brother Bill. I guess my memory was right.

3/10/01

Hey Vicki,

Maureen (and I) thank you for your letter. She hung on every word, especially when it came to talking about your father and the Scripture readings. She really appreciated it (and needless to say, so did I).

Funny thing. She's not always coherent when she's awake, but she muttered something to me about three days ago. She was pointing out that you and your dad were the first signs to her that Jesus was real. She said she could just tell from being around your family and that the impression never left her.

A good friend of mine died from brain cancer about a year ago. He kept seeing an angel up in the corner of the room for several days. Maureen had pointed up in the corner of her bedroom and turned to me with a huge smile last week. She was motioning to say that someone was there. Hadn't seen a smile like that on anyone since my friend's encounter last year.

If you want to send her more encouraging Scriptures, etc., please feel free. You can e-mail them to me, and I will go read them to her. ...

> *Bill*

Mom recently dug up a copy of the letter my dad sent Maureen during this time:

Dear Maureen,

Thank you for working so hard as a gymnast, which brought me happiness, and for being an inspiration to the other girls. You are a great friend. I became a Christian when I was 30 years old and have never feared death since then, even though I have been close several times. The death of the body is not the end for us. I'll see you again.

Julia Sweeney was on *SNL* with me. She did the androgynous character Pat. When she left the show, she got cancer. She wrote a play about it: *God Said, Ha!* Then, she wrote a play called *Letting Go of God* about her journey into atheism. I attended the play. She's a great writer. We hugged. We seemed to be the only two *SNL* alum interested in God and life after death, albeit with exact opposite opinions. But, to me, Julia's passion to not believe is maybe really a desperate hunger to believe. We debated God's existence through e-mails, and I sent her my favorite study Bible.

I attempted to write a responding play, *Holding on to God*. My title didn't have the punch that hers did. It didn't have the shock value. So far all I've come up with as an artistic response to her artistic public dismissal of God is a song called "The Atheist." It seems that atheists always act intellectually superior, a bit arrogant. So, I sort of played off of that.

"The Atheist"

She brags about her lack of faith
That's how she puts it
She sticks her nose up in the air
And says there is no God up there
She does not fear the Lord because
There is no God to fear
And she talks about it all day long!

She's telling everyone she sees
She's got the cure to our disease
Of ignorance, she shouts with zeal,
"There is no God, He isn't real!"
And she is now the master of her immortality
And she talks about it all day long!

There is no moral wrong or right
There is no black there is no white
She found this freedom, she has said
When she discovered God is dead,

As Nietzsche[1] said, "God is a lie,"
She likes to quote that German guy
And she's consumed with bashing
Every inch of Christianity,
She seems obsessed with Jesus
And His lack of deity,
And she talks about it all day long!

I say, "If He doesn't exist, why do you keep talking about Him?"[2]

Although it's not the reason I believe, many great thinkers believed in God: Copernicus, Bacon, Kepler, Galileo, Descartes, Mendel, C. S. Lewis, and Pascal. I do my apologetics in song, the only way I know how. I sang "The Atheist" on TBN in an interview with Paul Crouch Jr. around 2007.

The God debate between Julia and I became a public airwaves debate. We sparred a bit on *Politically Incorrect* with Bill Maher. I was on his show twelve times, always outnumbered by atheists. One time I brought my big Bible and plopped it on the coffee table in the middle of the room.

Another time Michael Shermer of *Skeptic* magazine was saying that mostly women believe in Jesus, inferring they were more emotional, weak, and uneducated. I responded, "Most of the people in the Bible are men, his disciples, the authors, etc. "The reason there are more old women in church than men is because all of their husbands died!" That got a good laugh. I quoted Ephesians 2:8–9 and the crowd, Bill Maher's crowd, his fans, actually cheered! God's Word is powerful and He says, "It shall not return unto me void" (Isaiah 55:11 KJV).

Can I prove there is a God?

I heard a teenager say, "You can't put a miracle in a test tube."

Faith is a gift. We can ask God for faith. We can ask God to reveal Himself to us. If He appeared before us, would we believe?

Jesus appeared to his followers, did miracles, and rose from the grave. Some of his contemporaries still did not believe He was God. His life, death, and resurrection were recorded by eyewitnesses in the Gospels and by the Jewish historian Josephus (a nonbeliever). Moses wrote about God between 1400 and 1250 BC. He wrote about the flood, the parting of the Red Sea, the plagues on Egypt, the cloud of fire, and manna. There were still doubters during those big miracles. Israel even made a pagan golden calf to worship when Moses was on the mountain receiving the tablets of stone, the Ten Commandments carved by God's own finger.

Faith seems to be a choice. An intelligent, personal decision. Creation reveals His existence, the Master Designer. The Bible reveals His Word and is archaeologically, scientifically, and historically (genealogies, kings, kingdoms) accurate. Jesus reveals God's nature—love.

In John 20:29, Jesus told Thomas: "Have you believed because you have seen me? Blessed are those who have not seen and yet have believed" (ESV). He also said, "Whosoever therefore shall confess me before men, him will I confess also before my Father which is in heaven" (Matthew 10:32 KJV).

TIP: Tell someone the good news. Have a good, old-fashioned fact-based, kind-hearted debate. Know how to defend what you believe in. Bible study, Bible study, Bible study. I learn something new every time I open it.

WHaT DID I DO WronG?
WHY IS GOD PUniSHinG Me?

"Neither this man nor his parents sinned,"
said Jesus, "but this happened so that the works
of God might be displayed in him."

JOHN 9:3

*M*y legalistic-holier-than-thou relative singsongs "Payday, payday!" whenever she hears that someone has cirrhosis of the liver or lung cancer. "They deserved it. They probably drank alcohol or smoked cigarettes."

That's not what Jesus would do. He said God "sent not his Son into the world to condemn the world; but that the world through Him might be saved" (John 3:17 KJV).

God warned that the wages of sin is death, but He knew we could not be holy. That is why Jesus died for our sins.

When I got cancer, I blamed myself. I just knew it was my fault. *God is punishing me!* I thought. Maybe He was. And, that spanking worked. I do not drink or smoke anymore, and I eat for nutrition, not to lose weight. But, I don't know exactly what God was thinking. "For my thoughts are not your thoughts, neither are your ways my ways, declares the LORD. For as the heavens are higher than the earth, so are my ways" (Isaiah 55:8–9 ESV).

I got genetic testing and the results were negative. The experts said my cancer was caused by chance, environmental factors, or lifestyle.

Then, I thought of the innocent children who get cancer, and then the Bible verses from the book of Job flew into my head. God said Job was "blameless and upright, a man who fears God and shuns evil" (Job 1:8). God let everything terrible happen to that man: loss of children, friends, humiliation, loss of wealth, sores, pain. Job said, "Naked I came from my mother's womb, and naked shall I return there. The LORD gave and the Lord has taken away. Blessed be the name of the LORD" (Job 1:21 NASB).

Hillsong's Darlene Zschech and famous paraplegic evangelist Joni Erickson Tada got breast cancer. They serve the Lord, all the time!

I wasn't a problem drinker or smoker. I was a secret drinker/smoker. I occasionally had a cigarette—every time my husband said he was leaving me, which was about four times a year. Once every three months. The pain of rejection would shake me to the core, and I'd decide it didn't matter if I lived or died. I'd get a stomach ache from loneliness and fear. I couldn't pray. I didn't know what to pray because my husband is a Christian too, so how could his God and my God have such different views of our marriage? My God wanted him to spend more time with me. His God wanted him to spend more time with his single cigar buddies who I call the Fornicators.

I'd get a secret cigarette from my secret stash, a secret bottle of wine, and go in the backyard to think about my options. Who would want to marry a woman over thirty, and then it was forty, and then fifty. A grandma? Twenty-five years of marital stress led me to seek relief in some form or other mostly food and wine. I didn't know how or where to get Valium or pills. I did pray. That should have been enough.

Then, there were all those stressful years in the late eighties in my dressing room at *SNL* where I was terrified. I did quote Scripture to myself. But then I had a few Marlboro Lights. But not in public. I was a Christian! I didn't want to be a bad testimony.

Can you get cancer from smoking if you're doing it in secret?

I had sipped quite a few glasses of Chardonnay when I was trapped in the Miami suburbs for twenty-five years. I was miserable there. I'd given up my career so Husband could have his career, because I was the perfect Christian wife and mother. And I reminded him of that every day.

I used Chardonnay to cope. No DUIs or anything. Just sipping. Lots of sipping. Jesus' first miracle was turning water into wine, but still, I felt guilty for this. God is supposed to be my comfort, not substances.

I felt even more guilty when the Internet said alcohol causes breast cancer. Though, in my group of friends with breast cancer, three of the five never drank or smoked.

To the church in Corinth, the apostle Paul wrote: "Or do you not know that your body is a temple of the Holy Spirit within you, whom you have from God? You are not your own" (1 Corinthians 6:19 ESV).

My eating habits were all screwed up. Since childhood, I was afraid of food because Dad, my gymnastics coach, told me I was fat starting at the age of five. I never wanted to try that first cigarette at the White Castle at Auburn University where that thin blond boy was trying to teach me how to inhale by making me watch my reflection in the night glass window wall. I didn't want a cigarette. I wanted a cheeseburger. But, I was afraid of getting fat.

Maybe cancer was caused by my lifelong eating disorders. Maybe plastic water bottles. Sunflower seeds?

I asked my oncologist what caused my cancer. The underwire of my bra irritating the skin there? Silicone breast implants? Cell phones? My friend Steph told me never to put my cell phone in my bra. I always stuck it in the left side, so I could find it. The Internet? Diet Coke? My See's Lollypop addiction? Not sleeping enough? Marital stress?

As I drove to each doctor's visit or removed each scarf or bandage or ridiculous itchy wig covering my chemo scalp that wasn't really bald at first, but more like a mangy dog with swatches and patches of missing fuzz, what I really wanted to know was: What made that one ductal mammary cell in my left breast suddenly decide to morph into a cancer cell? Was it the carcinogens in one drag from that secret cigarette? Or a buildup of them? One glass of wine or the cumulative effect of alcohol that battered the perfect cell God created and twisted its DNA into a satanic deviant form fit for hell?

"Was it … Ssssatan?" asked the Church Lady.

Satan is good at ruining things: music, sex, childbirth, marriage, families. My brother James told me there is even a musical combination called the devil's triad, tritone, or the devil's interval, the diminished fifth, that has such a dark side there is a rumor it was banned by religious authorities in the past.

Was it one stressful moment that changed that one cell? That time ten years ago I got fired from the failed Sofía Vergara/Joey Lawrence pilot on Easter, and I'd done nothing wrong?

I want to ask God when I get to heaven. I don't think things are accidental. I think there is a cause for everything.

Was it God allowing the devil to buffet me? Like in the book of Job?

Was it punishment from God for one of my sins that particularly ticked Him off?

Or are my ancestors at fault? "I the LORD your God am a jealous God, visiting the iniquity of the fathers on the children to the third and fourth generation" (Deuteronomy 5:9 ESV). Gluttony runs in my family.

What made the slow-growing cancer cell move to my lymph nodes? What made it suddenly get aggressive and move into nine of the twenty-six nodes, thus forcing my surgeon to cut out everything under my left arm and causing my oncologists to insist on five months of chemotherapy, radiation, and a lifelong estrogen-blocking pill that might give me perpetual hot flashes?

Did the cancer get aggressive every time my husband mentioned the D word or was it when I was sipping Bailey's Irish Cream liqueur and spitting it out so as to avoid calories?

Was it caused by the strange water at our mansion on the hilltop in Acton, California, that we only lived in for a year in 2009? That foreclosure house we got near the San Andreas Fault where I washed my hair, and it came out stiff? The water expert told us it contained arsenic left over from gold-mining days. We had to buy a $5,000 water system. Was that it? That house where I said, "Where are all the trees?" and someone said, "This is the high desert." And I said, "Oh."

Was it then?

Did the cancer get aggressive the day I found out Husband and the Fornicators, aka the Alibis (good name for a band), were planning a trip to the Keys on motorcycles to look at bikini models, and I wasn't invited? Or the night he came home at 2:00 a.m.?

Was it my tattoo?

God said not to get tattoos in Leviticus. But I was leaning on the technicality that we weren't under Jewish law anymore. Christ had come to fulfill the law, and we were now under grace!

Was it the genetically modified organisms that poisoned me? Monsanto? Cows and chickens living in cages and fed hormones?

Aluminum from chemical trails?

The Illuminati?

Did the cancer get aggressive the year I took the antianxiety drug escitalopram to help me not overreact to Husband's macho cop social life that continually excluded me?

Was it my broken heart that broke the DNA?

The Truth about Cancer by Ty Bollinger was recommended to me. It says cancer is caused by inflammation. And sugar feeds it.

Or did the cancer get aggressive the day Dr. Z., the dermatologist, looked at this painful spot under my arm and said, "I don't know what it is," and then took out a needle to inject it, and I said, "Why are you sticking something in it if you don't know what it is?" and he shrugged and did it anyway. Why didn't I stop him? I thought it would be rude, because he's the doctor and I'm not.

I recently called Dr. Z. and asked him what was in that needle. He said it was a steroid. Isn't that what body builders take to make parts of their body grow bigger?

I asked my oncologist Dr. Rexer, "How did I get cancer? If I know what caused it, I can prevent it from returning."

Dr. Rexer replied, "That's the million-dollar question."

I know that in John 9:2–3 when Jesus was healing a blind man, Jesus' disciples asked Him, "'Rabbi, who sinned, this man or his parents, that he was born blind?' Jesus answered, 'It was not that this man sinned, or his parents, but that the works of God might be displayed in him.'"

Did God allow me to get cancer, so He could do a miracle and heal me? Or show people how I trust Him?

He allowed Job to lose everything and suffer to prove Job's faith. Is this a test of my faith?

It feels like God is punishing me. "For the moment all discipline seems painful rather than pleasant, but later it yields the peaceful fruit of righteousness to those who have been trained by it" (Hebrews 12:11 ESV).

My family and friends say no, but I still feel responsible. And, I want to apologize to them for getting cancer and making them uncomfortable or sad.

I'm trying to get better, and not repeat whatever I was doing that made the cancer come. I drink Kangen Water I get from the local water store. I've switched to a mainly organic diet of fruits and vegetables, I take a spoonful of apple cider vinegar and black seed oil often, and of course, I don't drink or smoke. Although, my oncologist says he has an eighty-six-year-old patient who drank Crown Royal all through her chemo and swears it took the nausea away! I limit my See's Lollypops to less than one box a day. Also, I'm avoiding stress, sleeping eight to nine hours a night, and of course praying and reading the Bible a lot.

What is God teaching me through cancer? I'm learning to trust Him more regardless of the cause or the outcome.

Whatever is true, whatever is honorable, whatever is right, whatever is pure, whatever is lovely, whatever is of good repute, if there is any excellence and if anything worthy of praise, dwell on these things. (Philippians 4:8 NASB)

TIP: With the humility and gratitude of a guilty sinner having been forgiven, accept Jesus' free gift of salvation and enjoy your redemption. Then, try to be holy, just because you love Jesus. And, good luck with that.

DOUBLE MASTECTOMY: FLAT CHESTED AGAIN! YIPPEE!

> "Do not fear, for I am with you; do not be dismayed,
> for I am your God. I will strengthen you and help you;
> I will uphold you with my righteous right hand."
>
> ISAIAH 41:10

I spent the first twelve years of my life flat chested, and it wasn't a problem. I never even thought about it. Then, in seventh grade, all my friends' bodies started changing and mine didn't.

Doctors did many tests at the hospital and concluded that my extreme gymnastic training was postponing my development. Thus began my lifelong breast saga made up of many hours of mental strategy, trying to hide them or grow them or cover them or enhance them or reduce them.

Alec Baldwin was sitting next to me on the set in Studio 8H at 30 Rockefeller Plaza in 1989. We were rehearsing a sketch for *Saturday Night Live* and were waiting for something or someone. We had to kill time. Alec turned to me and said, "Why are your boobs so big?"

It wasn't flirtatious. It was angry-like.

I should have been offended, but I was flattered that he, the host, the movie star, was actually talking to me, the lower rung, the cast member. Also, I'm used to the direct and caustic manner of most famous actor types. Like, they use cuss words a lot. They have different rules than the rest of us.

One TV star kissed me on the mouth in Lorne Michael's office, in front of everyone, without asking.

One actor karate-chopped me in the back of the neck on the Vancouver set of the Nickelodeon show *Romeo* in 2005. It hurt. This was after he was arrested for having cop-killer bullets.

Another actor slapped me in the face once, for no reason, while we were on the set filming in 1984. I was playing his love interest. The grips were adjusting the lighting for my closeup where I was supposed to swoon, "You're so wonderful." Two others saw it happen, walked over to the movie star, loomed over him threateningly and said, "Don't ever do that again." True story. The show was cancelled after six episodes.

So, when Alec Baldwin blurted out this personal question, I wasn't overly shocked.

I launched into my detailed, chronological breast saga.

I know.

Maybe I was trying to match his rudeness and directness, kind of like sparring. (You don't scare me. I can be as gross as you.) Maybe I was just being overly honest. Oversharing is one of my flaws.

My breast history exhausts people and makes their faces gimp up. I have private photos of every stage of my breast development. Most recently, I have post-surgery photos of my double mastectomy. *TMI?*

What no one tells you when you are a young girl is that if and when your breasts arrive, they won't stay the same. They will morph into many shapes and sizes before they are spent and old.

My breast saga was very traumatic for me. I didn't have a sister, so I only knew breasts from culture, the beach, and my backyard. My dad was a gymnastic coach, so I saw thousands of developing girls in leotards in my backyard, and Dad took us to the beach. The ones on display were mostly perfectly shaped and sized. The old ladies on South Beach had strange ones.

I assumed I would get the perfectly perky ones that are on magazine covers. Because I was American, I didn't think I would get the *National Geographic* jungle ladies ones. So, it was rather traumatic for me that when puberty finally came (very late, age 21), instead of the awesome breasts I saw at the beach, I got sad little attempts.

Quitting gymnastics and gaining weight started my development, and a few years later I delivered two healthy baby girls, so all was well. Except my breasts never really arrived at the party. Well, they showed up, but it was a disaster. They could have their own feature film. It would rival *Titanic*. An emotional roller coaster. A breast epic.

Maybe I launch into my breast speech because, like my song says, I adamantly want the listener to know "I Am Not a Bimbo":

Just because of the way I look
Just because of what I wear
Just because of how I act
Or how I fix my hair
You think you can label me
But don't you dare
'Cause I am not a bimbo

Just cause my voice is high
And my attitude is light
It doesn't mean that I'm not serious
I read *Newsweek* twice last night
So why should I be
The brunt of your jokes, your mockery
When I am not a bimbo[1]

I am a nice person who was simply dealt a terrible set of knockers and had to go to tremendous lengths to appear normal in a looks-obsessed culture and career.

It never works. My long saga doesn't gain me respect but always makes the listener glaze over or melt into a face like they just ate a lemon.

Alec looked at me with a pinched face and then walked away.

At the *SNL* fortieth-year reunion, I bumped into Alec Baldwin again. We've both been divorced and remarried, raised children. He's done some high-profile work, and I've done some low-budget films. He fought for progressivism, I fought against it. It tickled me when he breezed past me and said, "Hi, Victoria." I'm still amazed that famous people know my name.

I wanted to explain to Alec why his socialist ideas would destroy America, but he was far gone before I could even respond with, "Hi." Maybe he was afraid of another breast story. I would have explained the evils of cultural Marxism/progressivism. You want income redistribution, Mr. Baldwin? Okay. Give me half of your salary from *30 Rock*. Spread the wealth.

But alas, Alec doesn't stop to ask me questions anymore. And I can understand why. I might have told him about my newest adventure—breast cancer. I might have told him my identity is not in my looks, or career, but in Christ. I'm a sinner saved by grace. I might have told him my newest joke:

> *Cancer hasn't ruined the romance in my marriage, because even though I'm bald, and my chest looks like it went through a wood chipper, my husband's a leg man!*

Maybe silicone breast implants cause cancer. They haven't been around long enough for scientific conclusions. I knew that when I signed the paperwork. I just thought age fifty-six was so far away. I had places to go and people to see, and I needed breasts to do that.

In 1980, I wrote this poem, entitled "Bust into Hollywood":

They said to bust into Hollywood,
You had to have a bust.
I said, "I must?"
They said, "You must."

Show business is all smoke and mirrors. Being attractive, in our culture, seems to involve a lot of disguise and trickery. God told us, "Charm is deceptive and beauty is fleeting, but a woman who fears the LORD is to be praised" (Proverbs 31:30).

First Peter 3:3–5 says, "Do not let your adorning be external—the braiding of hair and the putting on of gold jewelry, or the clothing you wear—but let your adorning be the hidden person of the heart with the imperishable beauty of a gentle and quiet spirit, which in God's sight is very precious. For this is how the holy women who hoped in God used to adorn themselves, by submitting to their own husbands" (ESV).

Maybe if I'm gentle and quiet and submissive, Husband won't notice my scarred flat chest?

Jesus taught: "But seek first the kingdom of God and his righteousness, and all these things will be added to you." (Matthew 6:33 ESV)

TIP: There are more important things than physical beauty. And, that's good, because I'm looking in the mirror and there's nothing to rave about. Kneel in front of the mirror and lift your hands and head up to Him and thank Him for your "fearfully and wonderfully made" body (Psalm 139:14).

SURGERY AND
THE GOOEY RECOVERY

But he said to me, "My grace is sufficient for you,
for my power is made perfect in weakness."
Therefore, I will boast all the more gladly about
my weaknesses, so that Christ's power may rest on me."

2 CORINTHIANS 12:9

I wrote this verse on the little chalkboard in my kitchen. I see it many times a day, and it comforts me every time.

After the initial shock, things move quickly. I am diagnosed on October 31. I have surgery to cut the cancer out November 17. Chemo is scheduled to begin December 28, less than two months after my diagnosis. On Christmas I will be woozy, suddenly flat chested, weak, and psyching up to allow poison to be pumped into my freshly scarred body.

So much information flies at me from different directions. Friends tell me reasons to do and not do chemo. Cancer-survivor friends offer me wigs, hats, and juicers, insisting that a blender is different than a juicer. Who knew?

I am given a special bra to wear after surgery, tubes to drain pus and blood that I will need to measure every few hours, pain meds, anti-nausea medication.

And I have a decision to make about whether to have reconstruction and what kind. They tell me about the DIEP flap that would take fat from my stomach and insert it into my chest, leaving a big smiley scar across my abdomen. Inflatable breasts could be inserted under my chest muscle, and the nipples would be gone, but I can choose 3-D nipple tattoos or other nipple options. I can't absorb all of this information so quickly.

The surgery nurse tells me, "No food or drink after midnight, no rings, no nail polish." I feel like I am going off to do a performance. I can't help it. I think that way. I always feel like I'm doing a scene in a movie. I've worn wigs and costumes before. I'm just playing a role. Cancer Lady. At death's door. Drama.

I am to arrive at Vanderbilt University Medical Center at 5:00 a.m. with lidocaine already spread on my nipples, which are to then be covered in Saran Wrap to keep the numbing ointment from smudging onto other body parts or clothes.

Husband jumps out of bed at 4:00 a.m. and is wrapping the clear plastic around the boobs he'll never see again. I take a picture of the boobs in case he or I ever miss them. I am fumbling my way to the car, trying to figure out how I will get the naked boob photo developed. Don't people go to jail for taking naked pictures?

I'm not that sad, because I've never been fond of my breasts. They are not friends. They are enemies. It is sort of a blessing that they are going bye-bye.

I hear my favorite radio guy and friend, Michael DelGiorno, filling in for another host and joking on the radio that no one is listening at this hour. I text him, *I'm listening! You're making me laugh! On way to surgery! Thank you!*

The hospital is just waking up. It looks sleepy and clean. I write *Cancer* with a Sharpie on my chest and point an arrow down to my left breast, so they won't scrape the lymph nodes out of the wrong side, if that comes to be necessary. The right breast is okay, but who wants a lopsided chest? Cut them both off. At least I'll be symmetrical.

I have gone back and forth about whether to get reconstruction. They will insert bags to inflate if that is the plan. At 4:00 a.m. I decide no. I don't know how to get ahold of the surgeon at that hour, so I write a big message on my stomach: *I changed my mind. Tell Dr. Higden no implants.*

Placed on a bed with a blue shower cap and blue hospital gown, awaiting the great drugs that will knock me out, I feel calm and optimistic. I trust my life into God's hands. He gave it to me. He created me, and He knows my future. He has my best interests at heart. Like the Bible says, I love Him because He first loved me (1 John 4:19). So, I sort of feel like I am in a movie, in a costume, and excited to see the next scene. A last-minute thought is to take a selfie.

Husband kisses me. He looks concerned. That's romantic.

I am out.

When I awake, my precious family is entering my recovery room. Husband looks a bit happy that I am alive, but a bit sad. He says something like: "They found it in the lymph nodes." I knew this means I'll have to have chemo, and it could have spread to other organs. Why hadn't I gone for mammograms and early detection? Because my mom, who is an RN, never did. I had no symptoms, no family history of cancer. Also, I had no health insurance until this year when Husband retired. And of course, as I told you, the fact that doctors are still only practicing! *When they get it down, I'll go! I'll go!* That's how I thought.

I am happy. Whatever these drugs are, they make me happy! My daughters are chuckling at my buzz. I am talking excitedly about string theory and how every cell is connected to every other cell in the universe. My brother explained to me once that an experiment had been done where they divided a cell, and one half of the cell was placed in Sweden or something and the other half was in America. They heated up the half cell in America and the half in Sweden got hot. Something like that. Anyway, in my delirium I am saying that the God particle they are trying to find at CERN—inside of a proton (proving the omnipresence of God)—means that when we sin, our sin touches God. It must hurt God so much, because He is holy and cannot be near sin. Deep thoughts ... and drugs!

The next two weeks of healing aren't too bad. The pain meds work pretty good. I have two rough patches from unrelated ailments. I get a case of vertigo, maybe from dehydration, maybe from too many drugs, maybe from the handstand I'd held for a preschool commercial I'd filmed two weeks earlier, maybe from turning upside down to wash my hair in the tub without getting my chest bandages wet.

Whatever caused it, the room is spinning for three days. That is bad. I walk to the toilet, smashing into the walls, then projectile-vomit and bounce my way back into bed. I can't lie on my side without the spinning starting. It is Thanksgiving, so my vertigo doctor is unavailable. I'd had this three times before, about every ten years. He calls it BPPV. He has a technique called the Epley maneuver, named after the doctor who invented it, where he forces you to lie on the side that makes you dizzy. It's all about an ear canal crystal coming loose from its little follicle and floating into the wrong canal. He makes you get dizzy until you're screaming and almost vomiting, then he hangs your head off the end of the table and rolls you to your other side, forcing dizziness until you scream again. He and the nurse hold you down until the spinning subsides. Then they sit you up and instruct you to sleep sitting up for the next two days. Once the crystal is snug in its correct place, you can lie down again. But, probably not do handstands. Weird, huh?

I also get a cough that keeps me up all night.

Besides those few days, surgery recovery is okay.

The comforting words of Psalm 23 run through my mind over and over as I make frequent trips to the bathroom to drain the tubes coming out of my chest that carry blood and puss I have to squeeze into measuring cups and then record on a chart. It seems comical, the ten bottles of pills on my counter labeled gabapentin (for nerve pain), Doculase (for regularity), ibuprofen (for pain), acetaminophen (for pain), lidocaine (to numb nipples before presurgery or port for needle entry), ondansetron (for nausea—it works), promethazine (if other nausea one doesn't work, but it makes you real sleepy), diazepam (Valium for presurgery), oxycodone (for pain—not crazy about it, I think it makes me dizzy), lorazepam (happy pill I could take right before chemo but didn't need to), Claritin (strangely, it helps counter inflammation caused by Neulasta, which is given to produce white blood cells in my bone marrow), omeprazole (in case of acid reflux) … pill, pill, pill.

All through the discomfort, and the inability to lift my arms, or lie on my sides, and those days of vertigo, and that cough that keeps me hacking all night until my abs felt like abs of steel, I keep repeating out loud and silently, and sometimes in song:

> Yea, though I walk through the valley of the shadow of death, I will fear no evil: for thou art with me, thy rod and thy staff, they comfort me. Thou preparest a table before me in the presence of my enemies: thou anointest my head with oil; my cup runneth over. Surely goodness and mercy will follow me all the days of my life: and I will dwell in the house of the LORD forever. (Psalm 23:4–6 KJV—the version I memorized)

After writing my first book, *Is My Bow Too Big?* I told my mom I wanted to write a follow-up book. She suggested, *Was My Dream Too Big?* I was thinking instead of calling it *Are My Boobs Too Big?* Mom and I had been discussing cancer and whether I had anything to say about it.

"There's nothing to say that hasn't already been said," I pointed out. "People should just read the Bible."

Mom responded, "But you're famous, and we like to read books, and you're a Christian." She was unpacking a box of two hundred coffee cups from her garage. When I told her she only needed two cups—okay, six for company—she insisted she was not a hoarder but a collector.

I told her minimalism is in.

I had just moved Mom from Florida to Tennessee to my neighborhood, so I could help her care for my ailing dad. Mom unpacked for a year. She has a doll collection and book collection and a thousand Santa Clauses.

I think I dreamed too big. I thought I could be in show business *and* be a Christian, loved and respected by the acting community *and* married to a faithful man who adored me *and* have lots of children *and* live in the Hollywood Hills in a nice house *and* do maybe two or three hit TV series directed by James Burrows *and* a couple of critically acclaimed movies after *SNL and* have a long, healthy life—*and* have perky perfect breasts. (Hey, that sounds like Julia Louis-Dreyfus' life.) I tried really hard to make all those dreams come true, but it's a broken world, baby! And then, there's the Second Law of Thermodynamics.

Now, I'm just happy if I can lie down at night with no vertigo, no nausea, and no coughing.

Maybe my dream wasn't too big. Maybe it was the wrong dream. My dream should have been to end world hunger and win souls to Christ.

The apostle Paul wrote, "I beseech you therefore, brethren, by the mercies of God, that ye present your bodies a living sacrifice, holy, acceptable to God, which is your reasonable service. And do not be conformed to this world: but be ye transformed by the renewing of your mind, that ye may prove what is that good, and acceptable, and perfect will of God" (Romans 12:1–2 KJV).

In the chapters leading up to this verse, the apostle Paul is talking about the wonderful, fantastic news that we were sinners standing condemned before a perfect, holy, and righteous God, condemned to hell, but that through faith in Jesus' payment on the cross for our sin and in His resurrection, we can have peace with God. We are redeemed, made alive again, forgiven, offered victory over sin and death, given the help of the Holy Spirit here on earth, no longer facing condemnation, but rather eternal life with the Lord. Paul then takes a breath and says that with all of those amazing gifts it is a reasonable response, out of gratitude, that we dedicate our lives completely to God and His service.

I dedicated my twenties to getting on TV and being a successful actress. I reasoned that this would bring glory to God. We need more Christian role models. But living a life devoted to nailing my next audition seemed to lead me down a few rabbit trails, like the fire-eater trail (my first husband) or the eating-disorder/"wine-is-low-calorie" trail—habits that weren't honoring to God. I had one leg in the world and one leg in God's kingdom just as we see in James 1:8: "A double-minded man is unstable in all his ways" (KJV).

Then, there were the TV jobs that began innocently enough, but turned into something a Christian shouldn't do, like the one where I played "Ditzy waitress who has a metal plate in her head, because a piano fell on her, and magnets and pens stick to her forehead." I thought that was hilarious, so I flew to Los Angeles from Miami to get that part. After I got it, the scripts became increasingly uncomfortable for me to perform. One day they asked me to hold an embarrassing sex toy in my hand and dust it. The next week they asked me to kiss a woman. When I said no they asked me to just appear to be kissing her. I said no. That job didn't last long. I didn't have to get fired. The show got cancelled.

❀

In his essay "Learning in War-Time," C. S. Lewis explores the conflict between a Christian's command to put God first and the human needs that also demand priority—war, education, finances, family, career, health, and friends. Lewis writes, "The solution to this paradox is of course well known to you, 'whatsoever ye eat or drink do all to the glory of God.'" He continues, "No doubt, in a given situation it demands the surrender of some, or of all, our merely human pursuits; it is better to be saved with one eye, than, having two, to be cast into Gehenna. In those special circumstances, it has ceased to be possible to practice this or that activity to the glory of God."[1]

In other words, sometimes it is impossible to live the Christian life successfully in a worldly career. One has to choose.

In his 1979 album *Slow Train Coming*, Bob Dylan sang that we all have to serve somebody, God or the devil.

Believers are missionaries wherever they go and whatever they do. They are either good ones or bad ones. I wish I could hear Jesus say one day, "Well done, thou good and faithful servant" (Matthew 25:23 ESV).

There's a certain freedom in being a minus seven on the beauty scale of one to ten. Maybe I'll work on enhancing my intelligence, kindness, and spiritual growth since my physical beauty is so limited!

The other night I was wondering how I could be happy if the end of this cancer adventure is being bedridden, skeletal, attached to a morphine drip, and bald.

I know how! I will worship God.

I crank up the volume on my laptop playing Nicole Mullins' "My Redeemer Lives" and sing it loud. This is what I will do if I can't do anything else. This is what we were created for—to worship our Creator. And, for all eternity.

I could pray too. I could be a prayer warrior and intercede for others.

Back to shallow, trivial, vain human concerns—my medical team asks me about reconstruction.

"Isn't that just psychological?" I ask the perky young surgeon's assistant. "I mean, I'm a grandmother. It's not like I'll be fooling anyone. There is no need now for lumps there. My attract-a-husband days are done. My breastfeeding days are gone. My TV star days are long gone."

"Yes, it's psychological," she answers. "It helps women *feel* better about themselves. Whole, healed, back to normal."

I thought I was above that. But, I'm starting to miss looking like a girl. Here's a joke about it:

> *"Men are visual," I hear all the time. I asked Husband, "If men are so visual and appreciate beauty so much, why don't they ooh and ah over flowers, paintings, and antiques? Husband said, "You can't roll around naked with an armoire!"*

❀

When I am shown the marvelous before-and-after photos of post-mastectomy breast reconstruction, it seems my choices are: (1) Cut muscle, insert expander to stretch scarred, tight skin, insert silicone implant (yes, they still use silicone though it's been tested for causing cancer); (2) cut stomach fat out, including the arteries and veins in there, push it into chest and sew shut, leaving large scar across stomach and the two across the chest with no nipples (3-D nipples can be tattooed); (3) leave chest flat with two lines scarred across.

I want the least Frankenstein option.

❀

After a couple months, when my surgery pain heals and after I do all my daily exercises, stretching the stiff chest and arm muscles back into circulation, I start enjoying sleeping on my stomach and sides for the first time in twenty-five years. (You can't do that with implants.) I like how my clothes look with a flat chest, although it seems to make other people uncomfortable, and I feel more like myself than I have in fifty years!

They tell me I have a year to decide on the reconstruction, since I have to heal first before they can cut me again. Who am I fooling? The only person who will see me naked is my husband. Will he really see the new boobs and think, *Oh, my wife is so young and perky! She must be twenty-five years old!* When does the need to look sexy end? Are wives supposed to be sexy at ninety? Can't we just kiss in the dark?

Abraham had sex with Sarah when he was one hundred and she was ninety. Very interesting. I bet their candles were unlit. Maybe not!

Dad told me all beauty products—lipstick, rouge, eye shadow, mascara—were worn to enhance nature, that beauty was simply the look of health, and that men were attracted to girls who looked healthy, disease-free, and procreation-ready. Even if men don't realize why they are attracted, these are the reasons. So, our fake white teeth, fake breasts, and fake nails are to trick men into thinking we are super healthy specimens perfect for impregnation. So, if this is the case, why would I, a grandmother, try to keep up the façade that I can get pregnant at fifty-seven? Is God still letting ninety-year-old women conceive?

Then again, it is polite to make our appearance easy on the eyes of others and Husband. It is respectful. I know it's my duty to please Husband, and it's a fun job. But breast cancer challenges the boudoir. When wives go through breast cancer, their husbands do too. We are one. It's his body, too, that is getting carved up.

But it's my body that is uglier. Scarred. Deformed. Not sexy.

I stumble upon these Bible verses: "Let your wife be a fountain of blessing for you. Rejoice in the wife of your youth. She is a loving deer, a graceful doe. Let her breasts satisfy you always. May you always be captivated by her love" (Proverbs 5:18–19 NLT).

I look up at God and say, "Now, how am I supposed to do that?" I guess I could do the second part, the captivated-by-her-love part.

FYI—miraculously, cancer hasn't stolen the romance from our marriage. It's still working. When our hearts and minds are in tune, the romance follows. We even did it during chemo treatments. I wore a wig!

And one of my jokes goes:

I can't do my shimmy dance anymore, but I take a Sharpie and draw little circles on my shoulder blades, turn the lights down, and turn backwards. I shimmy and Husband doesn't even know the difference!

TIP: Intoxicate your husband with love. No breasts required for that. Millions of other ways!

Start Chemo:
Poison, Do Your Thing

Yea, though I walk through the valley of the shadow of death,
I will fear no evil: for thou art with me.

PSALM 23:4 KJV

So, after my mastectomy and the discovery of some cancerous lymph nodes, the experts at Vanderbilt have a panel discussion about whether I should receive chemotherapy and radiation. They're on the fence about it, but eventually agree I should have it, to kill any stray invisible molecule of estrogen-receptive cancer that could still be floating around in my body.

Bummer. The treatment for cancer is worse than the disease.

This is going to be tough. Especially the bald part. God will have to carry me through this. From what I'd heard, chemo is horrid.

Chemo.

Suddenly, I'm intensely aware of a whole world of suffering people out there. I've entered the Land of Not-Heaven. I think of Mandy and her young daughter, Scout, who has had over twenty-seven surgeries for the rare Loeys-Dietz disease, and my New York friend Peter who was born with cerebral palsy and needs crutches for life, my firefighter friend Jim who lost one hundred friends and 30 percent of his lungs on 9/11 at Ground Zero. I remember my friend Mary whose son, Wilson, drowned in his backyard pool at age two. How do they keep on going?

I feel like saying, "This disease isn't me. It doesn't define me. It's

just a thing that happened to me." That must be what they are thinking and feeling.

I do my research:

> In the 1950s, an Italian research company, Farmitalia Research
> Laboratories, began an organized effort to find anticancer
> compounds from soil-based microbes. A soil sample was
> isolated from the area surrounding the Castel del Monte, a thir-
> teenth-century castle. A new strain of *Streptomyces peucetius*,
> which produced a red pigment, was isolated, and an antibiotic
> from this bacterium was effective against tumors in mice.[1]

Phosphoramide mustard, one of the principle toxic metabolites
of cyclophosphamide, was synthesized and reported by Fried-
man and Seligman in 1954. It was postulated that the presence
of the phosphate bond to the nitrogen atom could inactivate
the nitrogen mustard moiety, but the phosphate bond would be
cleaved in gastric cancers and other tumors with a high phos-
phamidase content. However, in studies carried out after the
clinical efficacy of cyclophosphamide was demonstrated, phosphoramide mustard proved to be cytotoxic in vitro, but to have
a low therapeutic index in vivo.[2]

Uh, so … should I take the poisons into my veins or not? Do you
understand a word of that?

So much love envelopes me when I start telling friends about the C
word. I e-mail Julia Sweeney, the atheist, and she says she is sorry and
that she is thinking of me (not praying for me).

Interestingly, my *SNL* castmate, Jan Hooks, dies this year from
cancer. *SNL* great Gilda Radner died from cancer, actually when I was
on the show, in the cast. We held a tribute to her.

My family is precious and protective of me. Husband turns into
Dream Husband for a while and pours love all over me in many ways.

Friends bring me food, send cards, and even offer to shave their heads in solidarity.

My ex-Muslim friend, who is now a strong believer in Christ, gives me a long lecture about the evils of chemotherapy. I study the facts she gives me and Ty Bollinger's book, *The Truth about Cancer*, and I agree that putting healthy things into our mouths is the best prevention, but I don't know that modern medical science is completely wrong about chemo. Four friends from my Bible study group have all survived cancer after having chemo. They encourage me to do it.

My health-nut friend warns against chemo. Joel Osteen's mother was healed of cancer without chemo.

Other friends insist I get chemo. "It's common sense, tried and true, the only option," they say.

My oncologist looks annoyed when I mention the conspiracy theories about pharmaceutical companies secretly hiding the cure to cancer so they can continue to make money.

Too much new information is bombarding my brain.

So, I go into my prayer closet and get alone with God. I made this prayer closet after seeing the movie *War Room*, to pray for my marriage. That prayer is being answered. Husband is spending time with me, and doing nightly devotions with me, and praying with me and for me. I feel truly loved by him, maybe for the first time.

There are Post-its and Sharpie scribbles all over my closet wall, my prayer requests to God. I add *Cancer*.

Yikes! That word stands out.

I tell God that I need wisdom.

"Please give me wisdom, Lord, chemo or no chemo. And, if it's your will, please heal me. Thy will not mine be done."

That phrase that Jesus prayed in the garden of Gethsemane, "Thy will not mine be done," reminds me of a song I wrote a few years back for my friend I mentioned whose young son drowned in the backyard pool in the ten minutes she turned away to say goodbye to the babysitter. I had no words of wisdom to give her. I asked God for an answer. I got this:

"It's Foggy"

"It's foggy," Mary said, as she slowly shook her head,
"You should see the mountains on a clear day."
"It's beautiful," said I. That was my reply.
"It's still beautiful, but in a different way."
Lavender and pink and gold, sunset's all ablaze,
Or lavender and blue and gray, Smoky Mountains in a haze.
Sun goes up and sun goes down, shorter nights and shorter days,
I wrestle with the will of God, but always I end up amazed.
Tragedy and harmony walk side by side and intertwine,
An accident, a New Year's Eve, a tall giraffe, the aftermath,
The carousel, the wishing well, the broken heart that hurts
    like hell,
A tear that slowly drips into a smile.
Children grow old, some never do,
I ask God, "Why and where are you?"
I see him where I saw him last. I can't go on. I miss the past,
I think I've lost the memory of fun.
But then I hear my Savior say to God on Crucifixion Day,
"Thy will and not my will be done."[3]

The next day after my prayer time seeking wisdom about chemo, I am walking into Panera Bread with Husband after yet another doctor visit (now I know what that male nurse I first met at the walk-in clinic meant by his wife *goes* to Vanderbilt) to have lunch with our beautiful thirty-year-old daughter when I bump into my friend Mandy. Her head is shaved in support of her famous friend Joey Feek. Our eyes meet, and I surprise her with my news: "I have cancer."

Mandy is shocked. She looks me right in the eye and says, "Get chemo."

Wow. "That's really weird you said that," I said, "because I asked God last night in my prayer closet whether I should get chemo or not. I was kind of looking for a sign from Him, and then I bump into you, and your head is shaved, and you tell me that."

Mandy continues, "Joey didn't get chemo, because she wanted to breastfeed her new baby, and now the cancer is back way worse. She's on a morphine drip."

I think that was God's answer to my question.

So I let the Vanderbilt staff put poison into my veins.

Now, why would God let Joey, the beautiful well-known singer of the duo Joey + Rory, have terminal cancer at the young age of forty, with a new baby? She is a healthy eater, grows vegetables in her backyard garden. She obviously doesn't have a sugar problem. She is a good person. She prays for healing. Why isn't God healing her? Why did God heal the four women in my Bible study but not Joey?

I ask God to heal me. "I don't doubt you. I know you can heal me. You can do anything. And, I want to know what you want me to learn from this. I want to bring you glory through this. But you don't seem to be healing Joey. And, you might not heal me. It's all up to you. So, why should I even ask for healing? But, I am."

I think I hear God whisper back, "This is your story."

I am to be given doxorubicin (Adriamycin), often called "the Red Devil," because it's very strong. Dr. Rexer suggests I call it something more positive. Psychologically, it will go down easier.

"Think of it as a good thing," he says. "It's killing the bad cancer cells."

I say, "the Red Valentine?"

Husband and I fall into a routine. Every other Monday we make the trek to "Medical World" and machines and tubes and life and death. We look around in wonder at the science and dedicated health professionals—so serious, so kind. I'm not really in any pain. We enter-tain ourselves before, during, and after the chemo visits. It's like dating! I actually kind of enjoy it. He brings me a Taco Bell salad, peanut butter cookies, and Chinese noodles. Not really healthy, but food tastes weird, so I have weird requests. The whole thing is a bit funny. After the poi-son is poked into me, we go to the movies or Husband drives sleepy me home. The Benadryl, intended to alleviate any allergic reactions to the chemo, knocks me out. I decide to keep a photo countdown, so I write on my hand with a Sharpie each week: *6 to go, 5 to go, 4 to go.*

Cancer inspires a new song: "It's a Broken World, Baby!" This song starts stirring within me when I tell people I have cancer, and they look at me like, *Well, how'd that happen?* or *Why'd ya go and do a thing like that?* Then, my friend's marriage ends while she is in chemo. That is all the inspiration I need. For a list of lyrics regarding broken things, I need only to use the prayer requests from my small group!

About this same time, my Community Bible Study group is study-ing the book of Isaiah, and we are smack dab in chapter 30, labeled in my Bible, "Hezekiah is Healed of a Deadly Disease." I don't remember ever hearing this story. But, it is more than perfect for this moment in my life. Isaiah the prophet comes to King Hezekiah, one of the few good kings of Israel, who respects and obeys God and does not wor-ship pagan gods. Isaiah tells the king to get his things in order. He will die soon.

Hezekiah responds. He "turned his face to the wall and prayed to the Lord, saying, 'Now, O LORD, please remember how I have walked before you in faithfulness and with a whole heart, and have done what is good in your sight.' And Hezekiah wept bitterly" (2 Kings 20:2–3 ESV). Then, through the prophet Isaiah, God said, "Turn back, and say to Hezekiah the leader of my people … I have heard your prayer; I have seen your tears. Behold, I will heal you. I will add fifteen years to your life" (vv. 5–6 ESV).

God then adds on a special miracle and turns time back. Reading this, I keep hearing Cher singing—over and over in a loop—her hit song about turning back time.

Fifteen years.

The other interesting part of this story is that although God promises King Hezekiah fifteen more years, Isaiah still instructs that a fig ointment be placed on the king's deadly sore. Medicine. I take this as a sign that although God is the healer, he endorses man-made medicine. As they say, He gave us a brain and expects us to use it for something.

So, I ask God for fifteen more years. I figure seventy-one is a good age to die, right? Better than fifty-six. I can see my grandchildren grow up. But, my mom is eighty-two, and she is not ready to die. Even if I got fifteen more years, it would go by like a flash, like the snap of a finger, and then I'd want more time.

Why are Christians afraid to die? There's a Bible verse inscribed on a tombstone under a tree in my subdivision. Amongst other tombstones of the family that used to own the farm that is now a bunch of identical houses, one says, Thomas Bond (1809–1887) and then, "For me to live is Christ, and to die is gain" (Philippians 1:21 ESV). This verse haunts me during my cancer year. It continually pops into my mind or falls across my path.

I don't feel at home living in a subdivision. I feel like a plastic toy person in a plastic toy village, a drone, one of the masses. Husband can't understand this. I feel like a home should be a special place. I feel most at home on Lookout Mountain in Laurel Canyon, California. That was my special place. Wonderful things happened to me there. I gave it up to marry Husband, my high school sweetheart, when we reunited in 1992 and went to live where his dream job was, Miami. But, even Lookout Mountain, my favorite place, didn't exactly feel like my real home. I think God puts a yearning for heaven in our hearts.

Carolyn Arends sings it so well in her song "Reaching," where she describes our tendency to reach for the past or the future or for more, when only heaven will satisfy our deepest longings.

The apostle Paul says in Philippians, "If I am to go on living in the body, this will mean fruitful labor for me. Yet what shall I choose? I do not know! I am torn between the two: I desire to depart and be with Christ, which is better by far" (1:22–23).

I would like to be an example of a Christian who is happy to die, knowing I'll be with the Lord and in a new body in a place with no pain. Why do we read these passages our whole lives and then not actually believe them?

Death has a darkness about it. It is not what God intended for us. "The last enemy to be destroyed is death" (1 Corinthians 15:26 ESV). So, it is natural to be uncomfortable with the concept. What did I used to stress about? Life and death are my thoughts now. No one needs me here. I wouldn't be missed much.

My husband used to joke, "If Vicki died, it would be the saddest two seconds of my life." Now, he won't even discuss my death. It's too real.

I ask Husband if I should have a funeral. Should I make a video of me singing and tap dancing, so I can perform at my own funeral?

Who would come?

My show business friends gave me the hand when I publicly stood up for conservative values. Then they turned their back on me when I publicly said it was wrong to have homosexual themes in primetime TV shows like *Glee* where little kids are watching. I'm an outcast in Hollywood.

I ask Husband who he'd like at his funeral. He says, "The people who loved me, who I loved."

I do a double take. "I'm not inviting them! The family member, T, who wrote that horrid text on my mastectomy day?! Looks like it's just me and the kids at your funeral, honey!"

I'm working on forgiveness. Okay, I forgive them. So there. They're still not invited.

"Love your enemies," Jesus said. "Bless them that curse you" (Matthew 5:44 KJV).

Okay, they are.

Unbelievers can't understand this joy that believers have and carry through any trial. We know God has our back and that "all things work together for good" (Romans 8:28 ESV). We "count it all joy when we fall into various trials" (James 1:2 NKJV), because we know the Bible is God's Word and "this light momentary affliction is preparing for us an eternal weight of glory beyond all comparison" (2 Corinthians 4:17 ESV).

We know Jesus died for our sins, and we are redeemed. We are seen as sinless in His eyes, because of His payment for our debt. We can enter eternity with Him—not because of ourselves or our merit but because of the price He paid. This is the gospel. This is the message of hope we are trying to tell the world of lost people, who can't understand it until God gives them the gift of faith. Jesus said, "Seek, and you will find" (Matthew 7:70 ESV). I encourage you, reader, to ask Him to reveal Himself to you. He will.

The gospel sounds like foolishness to most of my friends from New York and Los Angeles, but I still believe it (Romans 1). And, after all, "God hath chosen the foolish things of the world to confound the wise; and God hath chosen the weak things of the world to confound the things which are mighty" (1 Corinthians 1:27 KJV).

My chemo cycle looks like this: I get chemo on Monday. The Benadryl knocks me out, but the steroids soon kick in and keep me up and cleaning the garage all night, then the next day I wind down. Wednesday and Thursday seem to be the hardest days—I stay in bed very weak and tired, but the pills keep me feeling okay. Friday my body starts coming back, and by Monday I am good again. I get a week off to recuperate and then the next Monday, they knock me down again. This series lasts eight weeks and then Taxol is weekly for twelve weeks. Taxol is mild compared to the Red Devil, but it is cumulative and at the end of the six months, I'm weakish. I lost one pound and one of my chins, so I'm happy.

Beside watching old movies, trying to eat ice cream, and repeating Psalm 23, I play Debi Selby's rendition of Stormie Omartian's song "River of My Life" over and over on my laptop on my bed. I feel like Jesus is right there with me in the room being supernatural and reassuring and full of possibilities.

I try on different wigs and scarves, trying to land on a look that's me. I can't find one. The Raggedy Ann wig actually suits me best. It is how I feel inside—like a goofy, shapeless, raggedy, broken doll.

For the first time, Husband suggests a walk down the street with me. I almost faint. That's been my fantasy for a long time. That he suggested it is even more surreal. Walking in winter is a poem. It is snowy. Snow is magic to kids like us who were born in Miami. We are bundled up. He walks his weak wife down the street. I have to take a picture. I am feeling fatigue from the Red Devil, I mean the Red Valentine, and walking the block feels like jogging ten miles, but it is romantic. The air is crisp and silent. The snow is crunching. He holds my hand and walks briskly down the middle of the street, as if he is proud I am his wife, as if we are a little love parade. I ask Paul, "What can I do for God before I die? I wish I could do something for Him." Paul answers, "There's nothing we can do for God, but let Him love others through us." Great answer, Paul. He's good with those one-liners. We walk past the tree with the tombstones under it. I show him the Thomas Bond tombstone I'd discovered, with the worn-with-age inscription under the 1809-1887, that verse that keeps following me now. "For to me to live is Christ, and to die is gain." (ESV)[4]

In the Kroger checkout line, I'm reading the tabloid covers about Prince's death. The headlines say it was drugs and/or the Illuminati that killed him. I am deep in thought about Prince, his androgynous symbol, his catchy songs "Raspberry Beret," "Little Red Corvette," and "1999," and his Jehovah Witness religion. I am thinking about Prince's public conflict with his record label, his public mention of Chemtrails. I am thinking about the New World Order and the YouTubes I've seen of people admitting they sold their soul to the devil for fame. I am thinking about UFOs and how they might be the fallen angels/demons mentioned in the Bible. I am thinking about my pastor friend Preston who counsels people who are trying to leave the Illuminati and who have dissociative identity disorder (DID) because of trauma given to them as a child. Prince told Oprah that his dad abused him and that at age five he developed another identity.[5]

A Kroger employee, a pretty woman younger than me, is fiddling with the gum and candies behind me. "Breast cancer?" she asks.

I look over at her and think, *What? Who? Oh, that's terrible!* I have completely forgotten that *I* have breast cancer. I am waiting for her to tell me who has it. There is a long pause. Then, I realize she is talking about me. I have a scarf on my bald head.

I say, "Oh, yes."

She says, "I had it eleven years ago."

I smile. "That's good to hear." Meaning, *I like hearing survival stories.* A bond of love passes between us.

"It isn't fun," she says.

"No, it isn't."
She walks away.

I feel like Mike Meyers' SNL character Middle Age Man. A world-weary gravitas and a belly ("I'm working on it!") settles on a person over fifty, no matter how much one tries to cling to her carefree or slim persona. My parents are old now and need help with their cell phones; my children are grown and need babysitters and voting advice; and my immune system is weak and faulty. I'm wearing a wig, the curly, blonde one (but in public it feels fake; it's too perfect), and I'm trying not to eat my third Coffee Nip. The sugar urge is back.[6]

I used to work three jobs, go on auditions, and after an eight-hour shift in high heels as the cigarette girl, drink three Long Island iced teas and hold a handstand for sixty seconds in my stand-up act. Now, after my fourth chemo treatment of the Red Devil/Valentine, and the other poison I keep forgetting the name of, I'm so weak that climbing the stairs with Daisy the Maltese under my arm, after she's done doing her duty in the yard, wears me out.

My twenty-one-year-old is at the gun range with her fiancé, who insists she carry a gun to her last year of college. I'm praying she'll be safe. (The license plate of a suspicious car on her campus was traced back to a terrorist watch list.)

It's a different world than the one I grew up in. But …

Jesus Christ is the same yesterday, today, and forever. (Hebrews 13:8 NKJV)

❦

TIP: Jesus is the rock. Nothing can keep you down. Swim to Him and stand up tall and safe, arms to the sky.

Jesus is enough:
in my bedroom alone a lot

Lo, I am with you always, even unto the end of the world.

MATTHEW 28:20 KJV

*A*t my small group, Paula said, "You were at the brink of death. That's what chemo does, takes you to the brink."

Hmm. I was. What did that feel like? I felt really close to God.

Am I ready to die?

Joey Martin Feek died of cancer last week at age forty. She was beautiful, energetic, had a new baby. Her career was on the rise; she knew the Lord, and she smelled good. My dad is eighty-seven and doesn't smell good. His flesh is rotting. His back has bed sores. He wants to die. He lies in a hospital bed in the front room all day. He can't turn on his side. He can't sit up, let alone walk. He can't hear. The TV volume is on high and gives me a blasting headache every time I enter his house. Mom has to change his diaper and shirt and sheets every day. He hates his existence. He knows the Lord. He wants to go home. Yet, he is alive for some reason and not Joey Martin Feek.[1]

One has to shake one's head at the absurdity of death and life. God's ways are higher than our ways.

There are six possible outcomes to my cancer: (1) I'm healed and it never returns, but I eventually die of something else; (2) I'm healed but it returns in a year or more, and I die from it or something else; (3)

I die of something else; (4) I die in my sleep in the middle of a good dream; (5) I never die but walk straight into heaven like Enoch; or (6) Christ returns and I meet Him in the sky in the twinkling of an eye.

Does God have anything more He wants me to do on this earth? That's the real question, not *Am I ready to die?*

Bucket list: I'd like to spend some time in Italy, Florence, and Europe. It looks so dreamy. I'd like to write one great song, sing it at the Grand Ole Opry and hear it on the radio. I'd like to see my grandchildren get married. I'd like to see Austria and pretend I'm Julie Andrews on the mountain singing. I'd like to make a million dollars on my hit song and buy land in Leiper's Fork and build my dream log cabin and have dogs and flowers and stone walls and goats and horses. I'd like Husband to swoop me in his arms like a movie and kiss me for a very long time, without me asking, and then present two airplane tickets to Paris—no, Florence—from behind his back. I'd like to lose twenty pounds.

But, heaven is supposedly more wonderful than all of that.

Have I had a full life?

Dad says I've lived ten lives. He has a point. He lived the life of a gym coach in Miami while I lived the life of a gymnast, then a gym coach, then a typist, then a waitress, then a Bible college student, then I learned sign language, then I was a stand-up comic, then a struggling actress in Hollywood, then a gypsy/fire-eater/pot dealer's wife in Silverlake, then a New Yorker making TV money, then a Connecticut sophisticate riding the train to New York. I sang with Willie Nelson on TV—so that adds country singer to the list—a divorcee with money, a Miami cop's wife/mom/suburban housewife with no money, a Tea Party activist, a Tennessee grandma …

Seems like I've been blessed. I should be grateful and let go.

But, I just can't wait to see what happens next. I'm not sure there's any verse in the Bible that says people in heaven can see what's happening on earth. What will Weird Al's next album be? Will Aubrey have boys? What will they look like? Would I have ever won an Oscar-winning role in an important film? Will Husband stay faithful and love me even when I'm really old? Will he ever quit frowning? Will I be changing his diaper? Will he ever need me?

My time in Miami was like jail time. So let's add prisoner to my list of lives. I marked off the days in Florida as if I was scratching lines into the paint on jail cell walls. One life was my time in Acton, California, where I experimentally tried to start my career again, pulling my teenager out of her school and plunking her down in the high desert—making Husband commute every two weeks from Miami to see us. In that town, I was cowgirl. Add that.

Cleaning the garage one day, I found a scrap of paper with my daughter Aubrey's handwriting. She must have been writing about me; probably composing a poem for a birthday or Christmas:

Kissed the cheek of Hollywood
Waved goodbye to fame
Traded one dream for two others;
Scarlet and Aubrey Lane.

Those two little miracles made my jail time in Miami not only bearable but more than worth it. They never noticed that their city was crime ridden, swampy, and flat. They only noticed a mommy and daddy who loved them. We had a good life. A pool, a church, a dog, roller skates, bikes, dance and gymnastic classes, cheerleading, and birthday parties. Wouldn't change a minute.

Well, maybe a couple minutes, but not the ones spent with my two angels.

Some spouses of cancer patients leave them. Maybe they were going to anyway, and cancer is a good excuse. Or maybe it's just too icky.

"For better or worse." It's worse than that. Some spouses leave emotionally. Some read voraciously every heal-cancer book they can find to keep their beloved around one more day, because they can't imagine life without her. My husband was none of the above. I think he's still in shock about the whole thing and isn't really sure how he feels. Sometimes, I think he was happy that he might soon be rid of me.

Before my cancer, we were in marriage therapy, and Husband wanted to leave me. Why? I think it's because I'm over fifty. He might have told the therapist it's because I spend too much money. But, we live very modestly, and I only spend my own pension, not his! We didn't even know I was going to get a pension from SAG-AFTRA (the actors' union) until a year ago, because I never read the fine print. The acting unions had been taking money out of all my big *SNL* and other TV/movie checks my whole life, and now they were doling it back to me in my old age. Awesome. No one gets acting roles after age fifty except Meryl Streep. Okay, and Betty White.

A joke about pensions:

One day I realized what a pension is—they are paying me not to show up! Not to audition. They don't want to see me anymore, on TV or in movies, so they pay me to stay home.

Now that the chemotherapy treatments are near the end, Husband seems anxious to leave me again. He treated me so sweetly at first that I was happy to have cancer. For the first time, he treated me like a fragile piece of porcelain.

Those days are over.

I prance into the kitchen proudly dressed in my purple wig and purple dress, ready for my niece's sweet sixteen birthday party. Going to public places is always a challenge. I don't want to draw attention to myself at church, so I wear the Orthodox Jewish modest black head beanie. At the store, a neutral scarf thing. At a family teen party, purple! But the short one, not the long one—that's too sexy.

"Ta-da!" I say.

Husband won't turn around from washing the dishes. Hot smoke is coming out of his head like a chimney.

He's giving me the silent treatment again. Why?

"Tada!"

Nothing.

What did I do? Oh no, what did I do?

I start thinking hard. I did yard work, cleaned the garage, cleaned my car, helped my parents move heavy stuff, carried four bookcases into their garage by myself (even though I've been told not to use my prelymphedema left arm for any lifting at all).

What have I done? What have I done?

He glares at me. "Have you been taking money out of our joint bank account?"

"Only my pension. I need it to pay off my credit cards."

"I need that to help with some of the house bills."

"Well, sorry. I bought trees for the yard (fifty trees). And the *SNL* forty-year reunion (the plane tickets to New York, taxi, new dress, hair, hotel, snowed in extra hotel nights, rental car to visit friends in Connecticut, etc.). And then there's the bookshelves being built. I didn't spend it on cocaine or jewels or anything."

Shaking with anger, Husband sweeps the kitchen furiously and repeats over and over. "You need help. Unbelievable. You ought to see somebody. Unbelievable."

"I have cancer!" I exclaim.

I can't believe his priorities. He's snapped back into abusive Husband. The one that I suspect gave me cancer in the first place.

I must protect myself, so I pray: *God, please put a bubble of protection around me. Protect me from his hate.*

I remember all the old times like this. I could reach for a glass of wine to numb my pain or a lollipop to suck on. Now that I'm trying not to eat sugar or drink alcohol, I must pray. But, it's hard to pray about my marriage. I freeze up because God said, "No divorce." And, "forgive." But in these moments, the hate literally drills holes into my skin and heart and soul, and my stomach hurts and my adrenaline soars. I feel his hate. That's what he wants me to feel. It hurts.

I slowly gather my things and go to the birthday party alone.

He gives me the silent treatment for three days. Same old pattern. This makes me so lonely. I peek out the window and wonder where he went. I imagine he's at some cigar bar with the Fornicators looking at girls with breasts and hair. I can't compete with that.

Me and my irrational exuberance (that's how Husband describes my personality) lie in bed with Imaginary Husband. My pretend invisible husband. I show him YouTube videos of tours of the Holy Land and teachings on Revelation and the rapture. I like learning.

Back to reality, I watch *FOX News* and look over at our daily Bible reading book. We are three days behind. Husband is the spiritual leader, and he's dropped the ball again.

I open the book *Outsmart Your Cancer: Alternative Non-Toxic Treatments That Work* that my dear friend Connie sent me. Her boyfriend has staved off lung cancer for five years by reading this book and taking Protocel (not approved by the FDA).

I take my mom to the Gateway Church quilting group. I want to thank the group for making me a prayer quilt, where every knot had been a prayer for me. I had never even met them before. This touches me, and I want to thank them and maybe do the same for someone else. I want to learn how to knit and quilt. Handstands cause vertigo.

I sit quietly at the table of quilting ladies. They remind me of the *SNL* skit where the soft-spoken ladies talk on the radio with Alec Baldwin. They are calm and gentle women, so unlike the competitive actors of my past whose minds went a mile a minute and … well, whose claws were out. Jan Hooks comes to mind. So clever, so talented. This is what she said about me in the book *Live from New York*: "I just have a particular revulsion to grown women who talk like little girls. … And she's a born-again Christian. I don't know, she was like from Mars to me. I never really got her."[2]

Jan's biographer told me that she smoked and drank her Carltons and Robert Mondavi up to her last day. And, she sent a friend an e-mail that said, "Why is God so mean that everything that feels good is bad for you?"

I understand. I always thought if I got cancer, I'd double up on Bailey's, wine and cigarettes, and grilled cheese sandwiches and fly off to Paris for more wine and cheese, but that's not how I felt when it happened. First of all, Muslim terrorists are killing people in Paris now. But when I got cancer, I suddenly felt like I had the choice between life and death, and I choose life. Anything that was pro-life, I was after: organic food, cleaner water, more sleep, spinach, beets, carrots, more prayer …

Sylvia, the head of the quilt group, starts sharing that she is a breast cancer survivor, and so is another lady there.

I share my story.

Then, Sylvia says she was recently diagnosed with bone cancer, a side effect of the breast cancer chemo, and she is now in lifelong chemo for that.

No.

That is my next fear. A return in the bone as a result of the chemo. My oncologist said that was a possibility. The book I'm reading says that cancer healing by chemo has a 1 percent success rate and that chemo makes your cancer worse. Now, I have proof sitting right before me at the quilt meeting.

At quilt club, Sylvia prayed for my marriage. She prayed that Husband would not see me as a financial burden or a roadblock to his freedom, but that he would see me as a person who wants to love him and be loved by him.

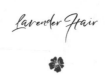

At my last doctor's visit, my Raggedy Ann visit, I asked him if I could quit chemo.

He looked surprised. "But you're doing so well."

I only have five left, but I showed him the thick book my Los Angeles friend Connie sent me that promotes no chemo and the holistic approach.

Dr. Rexer told me that some cancers just go away and that chemo is the only effective treatment known so far to have worked with my type of cancer, which is the most common type of breast cancer. "It worked in the 1950s," he said. "That's why they've kept doing it. And, I'm not in cahoots with the pharmaceutical companies. I have no connection." He added, "It has a 20 percent success rate."

Two out of ten? Scooby Doo's confused, shocked face here. *Aargh?* "Connie's book says chemo's success rate for cancer is 1 percent," I said hopelessly.

"Maybe that's all cancers," Dr. Rexer said casually.

Suzanne Somers made millions on her cancer books. Her hero, Dr. Stanislaw Burzynski, has identified missing peptides in the blood and urine of people who have cancer. He claims that antineoplastons, which are peptides, inhibit the growth of cancer cells.[3] But the Texas Medical Board filed suit against him last year saying he is a quack. So, who am I to believe? Somers had a lumpectomy and radiation but credits holistic treatments and nutrition for her sixteen years of survival.

I go to my prayer closet. "Lord, please don't let me get bone cancer and please heal Sylvia."

I have an idea for the quilting. I want to use patches of material from my children's saved baby clothes and sew them together to remember those magical days that flew by, when I was young, and they were young, and the world was young, and possibility hung in the air, and dreams could still come true. I start sewing my quilt of baby clothes and break Mom's sewing machine. Cost me eighty-five dollars. And, the quilt is all gimped up. Looks like a car accident of material. I quit sewing. I made a D in sewing in high school. That should have been a clue that my skills do not lie in that area.

"The LORD your God is with you, the Mighty Warrior who saves. He will take great delight in you; in his love he will no longer rebuke you, but will rejoice over you with singing" (Zephaniah 3:17).

TIP: Jesus is with you. Talk to Him. Listen to Him. Sing to Him. He sings over us.

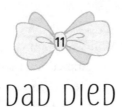

Dad Died

Whereas you do not know what will happen tomorrow.
For what is your life? It is even a vapor that appears
for a little time and then vanishes away.

JAMES 4:14

*D*ad taught Sunday school for fifty years. You would think his last days would be filled with angelic choirs, prayer meetings, a glow on his face, and joy in his eyes that he is close to meeting his Maker. But no, his friends had all died or moved away, his students were grown and gone. His loud TV was competing with Mom's loud TV in the adjoining room. And that horrid smell. I think his colostomy tubes leaked. Mom had the blinds closed from the beautiful sights of spring because Dad didn't like the sun in his eyes and because Mom thought she looked younger in the dark. She wouldn't quit dying her hair because Dad liked it blonde.

I wanted to talk about God, but even preaching can get weary when one is in constant pain. I watched my athletic dad lying immobile day after day. Pithy platitudes, and Bible verses seemed inappropriate in moments of urgent care, like when a rush of mucus spilled out of his mouth, choking him. I wanted to play worship music in his hospital room. God is bigger than this, but I couldn't figure out how to get connected to the hospital Wi-Fi. We could've sung hymns the old-fashioned way to comfort Dad, but we were all so confused and miserable. Doctors and nurses were coming in and out of the room, with helpless faces. When death is really coming, no one can stop it.

As Mary Steenburgen said in the movie *Parenthood*, "Life is messy."[1]

Dad wore his Gymnastic King sweatshirt to the emergency room every time he went. He wanted people to know he was a gymnast, not a smelly old man. (He was actually buried in it. A gift from Lisa Whipple, an old gymnastic student.)

Mom put their 8x10 framed wedding photo in his hospital room, so all the nurses and doctors would treat them like the people in the photo instead of old, invisible, unimportant non-souls. *We used to be young and beautiful*, Mom was silently shouting.

Very weird. But, isn't that what I was doing wearing a purple/gray wig in braids to visit them? Wasn't I saying, *I'm a hip, artistic type who used to be on* SNL. *I'm not a bald-headed cancer patient who's dying and irrelevant*?

It's frightening to think how unimportant we are. We die and the world keeps spinning. We aren't even a blip. We don't matter, do we?

King David wrote, "What is mankind that you are mindful of them, human beings that you care for them?" (Psalm 8:4).

But, God.

"An Old Stamp"

A little old man who lived alone
Saw an ad in the *Town Crier*
That said for a certain old stamp
There was an interested buyer.

He ran to the kitchen
And there in the garbage it lay
The treasure glued to a letter
That he had thrown away.

The buyer came over and bought it.
The old man was merry and glad
Though he couldn't quite understand
What value the old stamp had.

Only a square inch of paper
A worthless thing, needless to say
Whose value was not in itself
But in how much the buyer was willing to pay.

And so am I to God.
A blip, a speck, a worthless cliché
Who has no value at all in myself
But in the price He was willing to pay.

I am so important to God
That He left all the splendor above
To become a man and die just for me.
To Him I was worth that much love.[2]

I was hoping my parents would show me how to die with joy, with the Lord. Baptist deacon Dad screamed at Mom yesterday as if he was demon possessed, and I saw him punch her three times. She had brushed his arm too hard when she was adjusting his blanket.

But then, when she was leaving the hospital to go home to rest, he pleaded like a little child, "Please don't leave me."

When I asked Mom about the punches, she said, "He couldn't help it. He's not himself."

How will I die? Will I put on a show for the sake of my children and be spiritual and brave or will I fuss and cuss, miserable and embarrassed?

This is reality. Life is messy. Old age smells. And, dying is ugly. And it takes too long, sometimes.

I got a text. "Your father is in heaven." I texted my husband and daughters, "Dad died."

My dad died today after seven years of suffering. I am so happy that his torture has ended. He was listening to Elvis' gospel hits. His last word was my name, "Vicki." He was calling me in to his room to adjust his oxygen tube. He had quit talking about a year before. Mom held his hand during the final hours. As he requested, our family sang "My Tribute" by Andre Crouch, at the cemetery while they lifted his body up into the crypt. Dad loved Jesus and is with Him. My eighty-four-year-old mom needs me now.[3]

I had a vision that night that when Dad arrived in heaven and was greeted by Jesus, two gold pianos rolled up and *the* Andre Crouch walked up (he had died a couple years before). Dad gasped with wonder, and they both played and sang "My Tribute"! Then, Dad's gymnast Maureen approached him beaming and showed him to that all-gold gymnasium. Dad was beaming with wonder and joy. He spotted some kids doing full twists and aerial cartwheels. Then, I saw Dad in his new healthy body, doing back handsprings down the streets of gold, people clapping and laughing.

For those who love Jesus, death isn't an end but a beginning. "We are confident, yes, well pleased rather to be absent from the body and to be present with the Lord" (2 Corinthians 5:8).

Husband hasn't left me yet, even though I'm a minus seven on the beauty scale. When he isn't giving me the silent treatment, or yelling at me, he calls me beautiful, and he makes love to me. Maybe he needs a consistency pill.

I melt in his love.

My bossiness has been replaced with weakness and neediness. I feel fragile for the first time in my life.

God is no longer just a nice and noble thought but a strong presence walking me through the "valley of the shadow of death" (Psalm 23:4 KJV).

Christianity isn't nerdy and embarrassing, but a Shepherd with a rod and a staff who is leading me beside still waters, restoring my soul, preparing a table before me in the presence of my enemies, and anointing my head with oil. My cup runneth over. Surely goodness and mercy will follow me all the days of my life, and I will dwell in the house of the Lord forever.[4]

Cancer good.

I'm not having any big spiritual revelations, walking through this valley of the shadow of death. I'm almost getting used to being bald. Feel tired and weak.

I spend my days doing exactly what I'd probably be doing anyway, studying Isaiah for my Community Bible Study class, reading Victory over the Darkness *for my Wednesday night Bible study, studying Revelation with my Sunday night Bible study, and reading Carly Simon's autobiography. She is awesome, and she had breast cancer too! I almost met her.*[5]

In 1984, at 20th Century Fox, Bob Schiller, along with his partner Bob Weiskopf, were paid to write me a sitcom. It was called *Twinky*, and I was to play the ditzy but smart wife of the vice-president of the United States. They were the team that wrote *I Love Lucy* and *All in the Family*. What a different life I would have had, had that project actually happened. So many pilots (TV show test runs) disappear before they have a chance to happen. Studio heads change, people play politics—so many factors.

I was in about five pilots that never made it but could have: *I Married Sofia*, the 2004 Sofia Vergara-Joey Lawrence pilot; *Victoria*, the 1992 pilot written right after I left *SNL* where George Clooney plays my boyfriend; *Dreesen Street*, the 1986 one with Tom Dreesen that I shot when I was pregnant with Scarlet; and *Walter*, the 1984 pilot with Gary Burghoff (*M.A.S.H.*). There was also the 1983 short-lived *The Half Hour Comedy Hour*, and the 1985 short-lived *Half Nelson* with Joe Pesci.

Bob Schiller was always so kind to me. He was handsome and charming with his big intellect and white beard. He's ninety-seven now, still alive. His Christmas cards are always original and funny. He's a Jewish atheist as far as I know. There are a lot of those in Los Angeles and New York.

His son Tom is a successful commercial director and famous for his John Belushi and Gilda Radner short films. He did one with me and Jon Lovitz where we are in 1940s attire, lip-synching a love song on a balcony when a big wind comes and blows us off the balcony, and we keep singing and land on our feet below and kiss.

Tom Schiller knows Carly Simon. So, I'm only one degree of separation away from the wonderful Carly Simon.

Speaking of degrees of separation, which just reminds us what a small world it is after all, Husband hurt my feelings at our eight-week marriage class when he told the group that Melania Trump was attractive.

Always trying to find the upside to a painful moment, I replied, "Well, I touched Trump. I did a photo shoot for *People* magazine with him in 1992, and he touched perfect Melania, and you've touched me, so you've actually touched Melania!"

Christina Applegate and Melissa Etheridge are breast cancer survivors. Hoda Kotb had breast cancer. She and Carly Simon don't seem to talk about it a lot. They treat it like a hiccup, a flu, a cold that came and went, no big deal. I find myself in this category. I can't bring myself to read the ten cancer books stacked next to my bed, and I don't want to hang out with cancer people. I feel good and just want to act the same as I always did.

I did start googling mastectomy tattoos though, looking for a way to feel pretty without getting more silicone implants stuffed into my chest or the fat from my stomach gouged out and stuffed in there. The DIEP flap procedure requires a major vein and artery to be cut and resewn! Ew! Three months of healing and drainage tubes also.

A sweet lady at church who wanted to encourage me took me in the bathroom and pulled her shirt up to show me how happy she was with her DIEP flap!

I thought, *Hey, how about a 3-D picture of perfect breasts tattooed on my chest? Like a drawing.* Then I thought, *How about a tattoo of tassels spinning? Spinning tassels! Tassels in mid swing! Husband would like that, right?*

I'm inspired to clean my garage, which means I'm shuffling papers again from one side of the garage to the other, because I cannot throw anything away. I find letters from my early days in Hollywood: my family so excited to see me on Johnny Carson, my first paycheck from acting, a twelfth-grade drawing of my dream house and future children's names that looks identical to my current home and children's names, love letters from the one that got away.[6]

I stumble upon a tract by Anne Graham Lotz, who has the family gift of teaching the Bible. She has had heartache like the rest of us. In *Why? Trusting God When You Don't Understand*, she writes:

I understand that a turkey and an eagle react differently to the threat of a storm. A turkey reacts by running under the barn, hoping the storm won't come near.

On the other hand, an eagle leaves the security of its nest and spreads its wings to ride the air currents of the approaching storm, knowing they will carry it higher than it could soar on its own. Based on your reaction to the storms of life, which are you? A turkey or an eagle?[7]

But they that wait upon the LORD shall renew their strength; they shall mount up with wings as eagles; they shall run, and not be weary; and they shall walk, and not faint.

ISAIAH 40:31 KJV

Anne continues:

God allowed the storms of suffering to increase and intensify in my life because He wanted me to soar higher in my relationship with Him—to fall deeper in love with Him, to grow stronger in my faith in Him, to be more consistent in my walk with Him, to bear more fruit in service to Him, to draw closer to His heart, to keep my focus on His face, to live for His glory alone![8]

My faith is growing. When I lie in bed at night and think about the scenarios that may happen to my body in the next few months and years, my faith in Jesus is growing. He is all there is. When He is all you have, you realize He is all you need. I don't need an Oscar at 3:00 a.m. in the dark on sleepless nights. I don't need a twenty-four-inch waist. I don't need a more devoted husband. I don't need to live in Leiper's Fork. I need God. His Word is loud and strong, and it comforts me with its ancient truth. Its ring. Truth has a ring. You can hear it loud and clear.

I think of Joey Feek, who went from being a beautiful, healthy young woman to a weak, bald old woman on a morphine drip in one year. That could be me. Maybe a cancer molecule traveled to my brain, like it did to my friend Maureen.

I think of my cancer survivor friends: Debi, Susie, Cindy, Stacy, Mary, and celebrities such as Darlene Zschech, Joni Erickson Tada, and Olivia Newton John. Next year, I could be planting more rose bushes in my backyard.

I think of Dan Rupple's wife, Peggy, whose cancer returned five times over the last twenty years, and she's cancer-free today. I know that God will give me the strength to endure whatever the future brings.

God is more real to me now. And, maybe that is why He let me get cancer. It was an answer to my desire, "Jesus, I want to know you better."

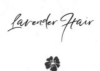

TIP: Soar around the room with arms spread like an eagle and sing, "When (your name here) waits upon the Lord, (your name here) renews her strength; she mounts up with wings as eagles, (your name here) runs and is not weary, (your name here) walks and does not faint. Teach me, Lord. Teach me, Lord, to wait.

FIVE MONTHS OF POISON AND BALDNESS

Now to Him who is able to do exceedingly abundantly
above all that we ask or think, according to the power that
works in us, to Him be glory in the church by Christ Jesus
to all generations, forever and ever. Amen.

EPHESIANS 3:20–21

*C*hemo doesn't hurt. And the nurses are so sweet. Although it is
weird that they are wearing hazmat outfits to shield themselves
from even a drop of the poison touching their clothes, yet they are
shoving it directly into my veins! I loved my chemo nurse Christine.
Her husband sold candy, and she gave me free samples. Sometimes
she wore a bow in my honor. Ironically, her husband got cancer right
when my treatment ended. And so did Fluffy Bunny (that was her
nickname). She was my favorite Vandy person who helped me with
all the insurance red tape.

Chemo isn't pleasant, but they've got it down to a science. I put
lidocaine on my port an hour before I went in. It numbed the spot
where they put the needle in. I ate, watched TV, and worked on my
Isaiah notebook while they hooked the chemo drip to my port. Nurse
Christine gave me five pills: benadryl, steroids, and some other pills.
No pain when the chemo went in. Side effects were expected to be
fingernail bed discomfort—strangely. And mouth sores. But, I only
felt a twinge briefly under two nails. Fatigue is said to be cumulative,

but I planted trees. I was pretty peppy. I was bald, so people thought I was in pain, but I wasn't!

So, I had my second of twelve Taxol infusions today, my only side effect to Taxol is a small amount of tingling/numbness in hands, a very dry mouth, and unquenchable thirst for a day. Thank you, Lord.[1]

Red Devil/Valentine was much worse, but there were pills for nausea and pills for every other little thing, so I have concluded that the word *cancer* is actually much scarier than the actual disease, at least in my case. The creepy part is that it is a sneaky snake that hides in your body and grows, showing no symptoms until, many times, it's too late and death is imminent.

That could be me. It could be you. We really have no control over much of our lives, although we live like we do. My prayer is that I will be dead to self and so devoted to the Lord, that on that day when he taps me on the shoulder, and says, "Today's the day you're coming home!" I will turn to Him and say, "Today? Really? Yay! You're kidding! Yippee! AWESOME!"

My ex-Muslim friend invited me to a showbiz networking party this week. It seems boastful to sell yourself, to list your credits, or to ask someone for a job opportunity. Anyway, it's necessary to find a job. It's also a great idea to get a roomful of people who have common interests together and just let them meet. So, I am psyching up to schmooze. It takes a lot of energy. But today, the day of the network party I wake up discouraged. It isn't the cancer getting me down, it's my marriage. Husband's love for me is unpredictable. It comes and goes. He is distant again, maybe looking for his next wife. It has always been an ebb and flow kind of relationship, but shouldn't there be more solidity and trust, especially in a marriage of two Christians? Feeling unloved in a

marriage is the loneliest life. Four recent events and a long his-
tory of marriage trouble made me text a friend and ask for the
number for a divorce lawyer. Divorce hurts worse than death. I've
been through it before from husband number one, the fire-eater.[2]

I lay in bed feeling sorry for myself. I was happy in my twenties, because I did what I wanted. I loved my career and my two homes in beautiful Connecticut and gorgeous Laurel Canyon. When I gave it up for Husband, thinking this was God's will, my life turned sour and dark. Leaving my career and moving to hot, humid Miami brought bitterness and regret. For twenty-three years I've been hitting myself in the head. Why did I marry Husband? Maybe because we had unfinished business from our college engagement that was never consummated. Maybe I was afraid to marry someone in show business because of the competition and instability. I don't know. Maybe I was afraid that other men would love the famous *SNL* girl, not the flaw-ridden, real me, and I didn't want a mate who would run when they saw the horse carriage turn to a pumpkin and my ball gown reduced back into rags.

Maybe I loved him.

So, after months of a good attitude about my cancer, my flat-scarred chest, and my bald head, the unending loneliness of my hopeless marriage is pushing me into despair. I cannot find peace or joy in my soul. I can't pray. So, I blurt out a disjointed attempt at a prayer. And Dr. Kent Robbins comes to mind. He has a daily video journal on YouTube about his brain disease journey. He ends each segment with a Bible reference and a prayer.

His struggle with a terminal disease encourages me. One night he said the way he is making it through is by the power of the Holy Spirit. The Holy Spirit, which is called the Holy Ghost in the King James Version of the Bible, has always scared me a bit. Ghost. Spirit. He's invisible. And He's holy. He's God. Part of the Trinity—Father, Son,

Spirit. When Jesus left the earth, he told his disciples he'd give them the Holy Spirit to comfort them and help them until His return. The disciples performed miracles with the power of the Holy Spirit.

I mumble to God, lying in my bed at noon, "Lord, please give me the power of your Holy Spirit."

I slept twelve hours, because I finally put my foot down and told Husband, "I cannot fight cancer with you waking me up at four to five every morning when you come to bed. It takes me three hours to go back to sleep, because you snore. And, you've woken me from my deepest sleep. I'm sleep deprived. For twenty-three years, you've woken me. You are not working the night shift anymore; you're retired. And, if you're not going to become a day person, sleep in the guest room and use the downstairs bathroom to do your hour of night grooming. I hear every toothbrush stroke and nose hair clip and *I need sleep!*" So, we've entered that old-age stage where the couple sleeps in different bedrooms.

I put worship music on my laptop. My bedroom becomes full of sweetness and light. I feel joy and peace. You can't dwell on marital tragedy or cancer trauma when the Holy Spirit is around you and in you. I think I feel the power.

I pull out all my wigs and dresses, humming hymns happily while preparing for the network party. I come up with a strange kind of Erika Badu head turban thing and I go mingle with my peers.

Everyone is kind and loving. And, I meet three cancer survivors there.

The next time I go to the Saylor Brothers networking party, I wear my funny pink scarf, because I'm still bald. I'm asked to speak, so I share *SNL* stories, the inside stuff, like what Lorne Michaels is really like. I say he's like *The Prince* in the famous book by Machiavelli: Should you rule by love or fear? He rules by fear. What was it like to be a Christian on *SNL*? I asked Lorne to remove me from a sketch that

I felt ridiculed prayer. He said he understood and gave the part to Julia Sweeney, who did it at dress rehearsal. It was making fun of "over-the-top" Christians who have Jesus salt and pepper shakers and such. No one laughed, so the sketch never made it to the live show. Also, I gave the cast the Bible on cassette for a gift one Christmas. Cassettes in cars were the new thing in the late '80s.

I recently asked Kevin Nealon, "Did I really do that, or was it a dream I had?"

Kevin replied, "Oh, you really did that. They're still on my shelf. I think I listened to number three and number sixteen!"

At this Nashville network party after my speech, a beautiful blonde, a former pop star from Croatia asks me, "What is your favorite thing to do?" and "What is your most challenging thing?"

Without thinking I blurt out, "Making people laugh and my marriage."

The most beautiful part of the evening was when the people with big credits traded business cards with the people with no credits. Jesus loves all people equally, rich and poor, famous and wannabe, young and old, pop star and cancer patient, talented and talentless. And, so do Nashvillians—they love everyone. God has designed us for community, and He blesses Christian fellowship. I have to fight the urge to isolate.

I've concluded that only with the power of the Holy Spirit can I face life's challenges. And only God can make my marriage beautiful. I will continue praying, even if my prayers come out clunky, unpoetic, and frustrated.

In John 14:26 Jesus said, "But the Helper [*Paracletos* in the original Greek] (Comforter, Advocate, Intercessor—Counselor, Strengthener, Standby), the Holy Spirit, whom the Father will send in My name [in My place, to represent Me and act on My behalf], He will teach you all things. And He will help you remember everything that I have told you" (AMP).

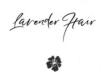

TIP: When you're down, ask God to fill you with His Holy Spirit, play worship music, and God will be there. He "inhabits the praises of Israel [His people]" (Psalm 22:3 KJV). While you are dressing for a party, wear something that makes you laugh. And then fellowship, not seeking a blessing, but trying to be a blessing. You'll come home glowing.

Handmade Purple Scarf

In the day of prosperity be joyful,
But in the day of adversity consider:
Surely God has appointed the one as well as the other.

ECCLESIASTES 7:14 NKJV

I have cancer. Cancer makes you suddenly aware of things like radiation and smart meters and microwave coffee/popcorn. Don't microwaves cause cancer? I tried to make coffee and popcorn the old-fashioned way, and it was a disaster.

Smoke Alarms

I awoke this morning to a piercing siren sound. I levitated from bed. Daisy the dog did too. All of the smoke alarms were going off simultaneously. I ran outside. The electric company man was starting to drive away. "Stop! Wait!" I yelled, running after him.

He stopped his truck. I think I heard him gasp as I approached, bald headed and in a black nightie with my leopard robe flapping from my arm and holding my traumatized, trembling Maltese.

"How can I, um, help you?" he asked.

That's when I remembered I'd asked the electric company to remove the radiation-spreading smart meter from my house. When they did, the electricity went off, which set off the smoke alarms.

"Oh, ha-ha. Sorry." I smiled at the poor man. "Carry on. Sorry about the alarms. Ha-ha. Thanks for changing the smart meter back to the un-smart meter ... I just don't believe the government should know and then be able to control how much electricity we

use. Ha-ha. And, uh, I have cancer, so … uh, the radiation is bad for that, so … ha-ha, carry on!"

He looked at me like I was nuts.

It was taking sleepy Husband a while to figure out how to turn off the alarms, and the piercing sound was permanently damaging my cochlea. Daisy the dog was inconsolable, her sensitive eardrums were probably exploding, so I grabbed some clothes and the shaking dog, got in my car, and drove off for a while. Hopefully, when I return the alarms will be off.[1]

Digging through my garage again (maybe I'm preparing for death), trying to throw something away, I came across a note in the beautiful handwriting of my friend, Glenn. His painting of an ocean sunset hangs in my home in a place of honor. We met at the Auburn University theater department. Here is one of the letters Glenn gave me in 1980:

I know a girl with golden hair,
She likes to count stars and believes in prayer,
She's full of life and sparks and fire,
And she's not afraid to walk the high wire,
Her smile is bright and appeals to all ages,
She's going to live life from a thousand stages.
I hope she lets me be there too,
So I can whisper, "I love you."

We didn't yet know exactly who we were or what we wanted to be, but creative things thrilled our souls. We listened to the eight track of "They're Playing Our Song" a million times in his VW Bug. I auditioned for the college plays and only got a line here and there until a student director, Becky, cast me in the British lesbian play, *The Killing of Sister George.*

In 1982, the year before I got on Johnny Carson, I had a breakdown and was staying at my parent's home, taking a hiatus from my LA acting dreams. I was about to give up. Glenn flew to Miami to give me a pep talk. He then came with me on a cross-country road trip, with my cat and its litter box in my car, to take me back to Hollywood "where you belong." He always believed in me. More than anyone. He believed in me before Crawford, Carson, and Lorne. He made me believe in myself. I believe in him too.

He's a wonderful screenwriter, and he's sensitive, observant, curious, and classy, with a Southern gentlemen's gentleness and drawl. He's from Atlanta. He knows Hoda Kotb. He used to work with her at the same TV news station in New Orleans. I want him to write me an Oscar role for my golden years.

I haven't seen Glenn in six years. He's a TV News Producer in LA now. During our last lunch at Jerry's Deli in Studio City, we confessed our secret sins to each other. He had just dyed a touch of purple into his hair and said he dreamt about me last night.

I sent him the bald picture I took with my grandchild. In it, I'm showing the thin, deep purple scarf he knitted and sent me when he heard I had cancer. His attached note said, "I made this to go with your lovely lavender wig. I hope it will bring you warmth and wrap you with my love."

"Two are better than one, because they have a good return for their labor: If either of them falls down, one can help the other up. But pity anyone who falls and has no one to help them up" (Ecclesiastes 4:9–10).

TIP: Don't wait for cancer to look up old friends. Friends are gifts from God. God is love. "Every good and perfect gift is from above, coming down from the Father of the heavenly lights, who does not change like shifting shadows" (James 1:17). Glenn is that friend for me, a true gift from God.

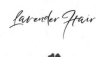

I spy on Husband's cell. I have to. He doesn't tell me anything. On November 17, the day my breasts were getting sliced off, chopped up, and thrown into a pail, taken to a lab and sliced some more to look at under a microscope, my husband's family member, T, texted him: "Isn't it funny that these well-meaning idiots (curse word) don't have a clue what you're really thinking? Hey, when this nightmare's over, meet me at the farm. I'll drive. Bringing scotch. Love you."[3]

Wow. What does this mean? I'm looking at this text. It breaks my heart. The intimacy and friendship with Husband I had been praying for now seems like a complete impossibility. Our marriage that was hanging by a thread is now hanging by an invisible reduced-sheen polyester monofilament.

I used to despise the bad influences in Husband's life and criticize him for his friendships while scolding, pouting, and sometimes yelling. That didn't fix anything. My new solution in this matter is to pray for them.

One day, someone in my Bible study class said that Christians don't have to be happy when bad things are happening. I thought she was referring to the "irrational exuberance" photo taken at my fourth chemo appointment, which is being passed around on Facebook. I took it as a scolding or a finger wagging.

So, here's a sad moment for her. My ninth chemo was the first time I was at chemo alone. I asked Husband not to come.

I cannot take stress into my fragile body. I'm willing calmness. Serenity now. So, for that Christian in my Bible study class who insists that Christians don't always need to be happy, I will add a sad chemo picture to the book. I can be sad.

I can't help it, but my default face is happy. I named my first stuffed dog Happy. I actually feel so healthy. Maybe because five to ten years of cancer growth was cut out of me. It feels in my insides like I'm clean and new. I look at pictures from the past ten years, and I was bloated and unhealthy looking. There is also a strange euphoria when walking through the valley of the shadow of death. Each day is special and new.

I also believe that dying will be a wonderful thing. So, excuse my joy. It must look weird.

I also like being flat chested. A huge load is gone. Carrying around all that weight. And, bald is expanding my horizon to new looks. I feel like everything is new.

I've noticed that I'm gradually returning to sugar, not my nightly lollipop habit, but along with my strange cravings (like for citrus—I ate eight grapefruit one day), I've begun eating waffles with syrup, ice cream, cookies, etc. Oh, wretched soul that I am!

My vet, Dr. Crowell, who fixed little old Daisy the Maltese's tooth problem, called me to express his concern for my health. He remarked that he's noticed an increase in breast cancer in his animal patients' owners in our area. His scientific training has led him to the conclusion that it might be the plastic water bottles, that when heated in the sun or storage, leak plastic into the water. He said that plastic is an estrogen simulator. Having a wife and two daughters has led him to keep his family drinking water only out of glass.[4]

That water craze. I remember when it began. I was auditioning for a movie. Lea Thompson, the actress, was sitting next to me at the audition. She had a large plastic bottle of water in her purse and she was sipping from it. She had the perfect face, hair, and figure. The water! It must be the secret to movie star beauty. Suddenly, I noticed plastic water bottles for sale everywhere.

I think there hasn't been a day since that day in 1988 that I haven't drunk more than two plastic bottles of water a day, thinking I was doing something healthy.

So, I googled it and found this on breastcancer.org:

> BPA is a weak synthetic estrogen found in many rigid plastic products, food and formula can linings, dental sealants, and on the shiny side of paper cashier receipts (to stabilize the ink). Its estrogen-like activity makes it a hormone disruptor, like many other chemicals in plastics. Hormone disruptors can affect how estrogen and other hormones act in the body, by blocking them or mimicking them, which throws off the body's hormonal balance. Because estrogen can make hormone-receptor-positive breast cancer develop and grow, many women choose to limit their exposure to these chemicals that can act like estrogen.[5]

I woke up one morning dreaming that I was at *SNL*, full of adrenalin. It was my last show, and I had to think of something really good for the Update Desk. When I asked Al Franken for ideas, he was dressed as Mick Jagger, and he said, "How about a movie review. Those are always funny." I was trying to think of the last movie I saw and how to make it a funny review. Then, I woke up and realized my last *SNL* show was twenty-four years ago. Oh yeah. What was my last sketch? Oh yeah, I did a handstand on the Update Desk with "I Love a Cop" on my legs, and I was singing the theme from the Broadway musical *I Love a Cop*. I think Joanne Worley from *Laugh In* gave me that idea when I bumped into her in New York. That *SNL* adrenaline experience never leaves me. *SNL* now lives in my dreams.

Wearing my favorite purple wig, I waltzed into Vanderbilt for my weekly infusion of terrific Taxol. Husband was with me. We had discussed my broken heart and the horrid text from T, which I photographed with my cell and tucked away in my Bible to deal with at a later time. I'm fighting cancer now.

My daughter called and said, "What'ya doin?"

I replied, "Getting poisoned to death."

They took my blood. Then, I saw my oncologist, Dr. Rexer. I love him because he laughs at my jokes.

I said to him, "It must be icky to see middle-aged cancer women all day. Are any of them sad? I'm not. I haven't taken any of that Ativan or antianxiety medication, because I'm feeling so happy."

Dr. Rexer replied sadly, "Well, some of them, when it returns."

"Oh … yeah. That." I said. "So, we do all this chemo, radiation, *blah, blah, blah*, and hope it doesn't return, and if it does, we do chemo again and again until our bodies can't take it anymore and then we do the morphine drip and die?"

Dr. Rexer chuckled awkwardly. "Well, we're working on getting you healed and it not returning."

I told him, "I hope it doesn't return in my brain."

Husband said, "Those cancer cells will die from exhaustion long before they can locate something that small."

Funny.

Jokes from my act:

There's a lot of crime in Miami, that's why Paul likes it there. (laugh) Once we were driving along and the car next to us had really scary looking guys in it. I said, "Paul, that car next to us has hoodlums in it." Paul said, "Vicki, they can read your lips." I said, "Oh no, they could shoot my brains out." (laugh) Paul said, "It would take some marksman to hit that BB." (laugh)

Once we took that Chuck Colson course at church, How Now Shall We Live? *It had hard stuff about Neitzche and Darwin. I said, "Paul, my brain is going to explode." Paul said, "If you're brain exploded, it would sound like this: pfft." (laugh) I said, "Oh, that's good, how do you spell* pfft?" *(laugh)*

I like it. He's flirting with me.

Paul used to come home from work in his little police cos-
tume. (laugh) I like to call it that because he takes it "so seriously."
Bang bang, 10–4, I had a perimeter, chased a vehicle, perime-
ter, perpetrator, canine, affirmative, safety belt (laugh) … I think
he uses big words because tax payers are paying and it makes it
sound more important because mostly the cops just show up after
the crime and wrap yellow tape around it. (laugh) No, I think
he uses big words really because he's threatened by my intellect.
(laugh) He knows that I skipped second grade. But he says every-
thing you need to know you learn in second grade. (laugh) And,
he knows that when I was twelve my dad took me to the Univer-
sity of Miami for an IQ test and they wouldn't give us the score
because they said it would affect our lives forever. (laugh)

Paul really looks like the perfect husband. He does chemo with me,
goes to church and Bible studies with me, has never owned a *Playboy*
magazine, does all the grocery shopping, all the laundry, cooks, cleans
the bathrooms, and tells me I'm pretty even when I'm a minus seven
on a scale of one to ten.

But, sometimes he hurts me so bad. And, by the way, cleaning the
toilet isn't my love language. I'd rather he write love songs for me on
the piano all day.

More jokes:

And, we are so opposite.
Husband says he wants to go through life invisible and when
he dies, people say, "Who was that guy?!" My motto is, "I WILL
NOT BE IGNORED!" (laugh)

I asked Dr. Rexer about the plastic water bottles. He said, "There is
no science proving that. BPA-free plastic is all the rage now."

I forgot to ask him about chlorinated tap water, which my one
friend insisted is the cause of cancer.

Another friend says it's the fake food, fast food, and the chemicals in our food. Some say that the fake estrogen in the food is making men turn feminine.

Dr. Rexer and his assistant liked my purple wig. I told them I don't know how to top that for my next visit. They don't realize they're my audience now, and I value their smiles as much as I valued Lorne Michaels' and America's when I was on *SNL*. I recently asked God if I could go back into the comedy world in some fashion. I don't like all this serious stuff.

I'm thinking a one-woman comedy show called *It's a Broken World, Baby!*, which explains biblically where human suffering came from and why we have it and the future of suffering:

1. Started in garden of Eden when Adam and Eve disobeyed God and didn't believe His Word.
2. The Second Law of Thermodynamics, which says the world is in a state of entropy, broken, getting worse not better. A result of sin. (Evolution is an unproven theory that ignores the above law.)
3. Sin must be paid for by blood. "Without shedding of blood there is no remission ..." (Hebrews 9:22 KJV). Thus, we have the Old Testament animal sacrifices and then the Lamb—Jesus. God is holy. Sin separates us from Him. We all deserve hell for our sins. Jesus took our place on the cross. "But He was wounded for our transgressions, He was bruised for our iniquities; the chastisement for our peace was upon Him; and by His stripes we are healed. All we like sheep have gone astray; we have turned, every one, to his own way; and the LORD has laid on Him the iniquity of us all" (Isaiah 53:5–6 KJV).
4. Jesus said, "If anyone would come after me, let him deny himself and take up his cross and follow me" (Matthew

16:24 ESV). "If the world hates you, know that it has hated me before it hated you" (John 15:18 ESV). When Jesus' followers suffer, it is our most powerful testimony, because our true colors are most visible when we are in pain, when our defenses and pretenses—hair and boob—are gone and our soul is naked before the world.

5. As we follow Christ, mature as Christians, grow in the faith, are being sanctified, and start to look/act more like Jesus, we die to self and live for Him. We live every day asking Him what we can do to spread the gospel, love others, and serve Him.

6. So, when He taps us on the shoulder one day and says, "Today, you're going home." We don't say, "Oh bummer!" We say, "Awesome!"

Wait a minute! That's not a one-woman comedy show! That's a sermon!

I wore my purple wig to the movies to see *Risen*. I was recognized by a young popcorn salesman who was born four years after I left *SNL* to raise my family. Maybe he saw reruns or recognized me because I'm wearing a wig. I wore a lot of wigs on TV.

Risen stuck in my head and made me understand my faith better than I ever have.

I keep thinking about the scene where the Roman centurion sits alone with Jesus on top of the mountain under the stars, and Jesus asks him, "What do you want?" There's a pause. And then, in the guy's own words that he'd said earlier when Jesus wasn't near him, Jesus answers, "You want a day with no death. And peace."

What would I say if Jesus asked me that? To lose twenty pounds, or that $600 leopard doggie canopy bed I saw in *Spoiled Doggie* magazine, or the ceiling-to-floor bookshelves I've been dreaming of putting in my jungle room with the big screen TV and the real lion rug, or more money for the Compassion International kids and maybe the opportunity to meet them in person, or the cure for cancer? If I could only answer one thing, I think my deepest wish would be no death and peace for everyone.

I asked Dr. Rexer if I could have a glass of wine when this whole cancer thing was over. He said, "Any amount of alcohol is adding to the possibility of growing your cancer, and any amount of alcohol you don't drink is helping you fight the possibility of your cancer returning. We have tested that."

Well. All righty then. Looks like God ran out of patience with His subtle hints at telling me to cut back on the Chardonnay, and now He's using the heavy artillery—cancer—to rip that Kendall Jackson bottle out of my hands. Scared straight.

I asked Dr. Rexer, "So you think a bottle of wine a night is a lot?"

He looked a little surprised. "How big is the bottle?"

"You know, a bottle, four glasses, but spread out."

"Yes. That is too much. You drank that much every night?"

I calmly replied, "Yes. Well, it was mostly just sipping. I hated living in Miami and could not endure it. I was trapped there for twenty years for Husband's job. Every night for twenty years I sipped one glass of wine from 6:00 p.m. to 7:00 p.m., as I cooked dinner—"

Husband interjected, "You cooked?"

I calmly continued, "Yes. I cooked spinach for the kids every night. (Put Parmesan on it to trick them into eating a dark green vegetable.) Then, I sipped a glass from seven to eight and helped them with homework, then sipped one from eight to nine as I tucked them in, sang and read, kissed and prayed. Then I sipped one from nine to ten as I watched actors who I used to beat out for roles doing TV shows I couldn't audition for anymore, because I was held captive in the suburbs. Then I sipped one glass from ten to eleven as I laid in bed alone, because Cop Husband was at work every night until 5:00 a.m., smoking cigars and laughing with his carnal friends in the hangar and taking them and their hot girlfriends on free police helicopter rides as I sat alone watching the Bible Channel, so I wouldn't cry. Then I sipped another glass of wine from eleven to twelve. Because I was crying."

I wasn't hanging from chandeliers or anything.

Husband interrupted, "I don't think the doctor wants to hear about your—"

"This is science!" I said assertively. "They need this for scientific research for future patients, for pie charts and graphs and stuff! Then Husband would crash the door open at 5:00 a.m., making the dogs start barking. Then he did his night grooming until 5:50, and right when I started to drift off to sleep, the alarm rang, and I got up at 6:00 a.m. and drove the kids to school."

That is my justification for my love affair with Chardonnay. It was not a careless or irresponsible choice.

I wish wine and cigarettes and cheese and lollipops were not unhealthy. They do help numb pain. But, I should find my comfort, my crutch, in Jesus, not in substances. I should.

I think Dr. Rexer made a mental note to add this new wine revelation to my chart. Secrets come out when death is near.

Today, I'm finally brave enough to look at my Facebook and see the comments under my "I Have Cancer!" announcement to the world. I teared up at the loads of loving comments from strangers and friends. Their kindness poured over me like a velvet cloud. One guy said, "You don't deserve this." One said, "You don't know how loved you are." Two were hateful, so I went to their Facebook pages. I responded, "I'm praying for you. I sense a lot of anger. God is love. And, He loves you and so do I."

I took screenshots to save the comments. Maybe I'll ponder them the next time I get disgruntled with life like when Husband is at the cigar bar, which I can't go to, because I have cancer and can't breathe smoke!

❀

So I'm sitting in my chemo chair behind a curtain, in my purple/gray wig, watching American Idol *reruns on my laptop, with my ear buds (to vicariously experience the highs and lows of auditioning, which I miss). Next to me is my sexy, perfect-body-works-out-every-day muscle man husband who could snag a twenty-year-old wife in a second, and when I die he can keep her happy with my SAG/AFTRA pension added to his cop pension! Husband watches* Dateline's *murder mysteries every day, but he needn't plot my death to get rich, I'm dying of cancer! Lucky him.*

So, Husband is sitting next to me, watching his daily murder fix on the hospital TV, the bloodier, the grislier the better, and in walks Pet Therapy Lady, a twenty-five-year-old brunette with a golden lab. Once a week she volunteers at the hospital, to bring dog-love to the ugly, middle-aged, boob-less, bald chemo patients like me.

"Layla, sit," she says.

Yes, Layla, as in [Bob Dylan's 1967 song] "Lay Lady Lay." ... Layla's owner has great hair and a great body just like Layla. Layla's owner continues talking to Husband for twenty minutes, oohing and ahing about the canine unit at his ex-cop career, his chopper, his guns, his muscles. Then Layla, who like her Master never glances at me once to comfort me, does her three dog tricks: shake, sit, and sit up, for her dog treat. I give Dog Lady a few mean looks and she leaves. Husband watches Pet Therapy Lady's derriere wistfully as she sashays her goodwill and her dog down the corridor. And I think loudly, Thanks a lot, Pet Therapy Lady—you are the reason I have cancer. Please don't comfort me next week. Please. I have a dog, and she actually calms me, licks me, nuzzles me, and assures me of healing.

Actually, my dog worships me. I'll tape a sign on Daisy that says, "Pet Therapy" and bring her next week.[6]

I promptly write a song about how I feel like a dog who is loyal and true to a master who doesn't appreciate me:

"Like a Dog"

Why did I never leave?
Why did I always stay?
Why did I run and hide
When you looked at me that way?
Why did I wait for you
When you were out all night?
Because I loved you like a dog
(loyal and true)
Because I loved you like a dog
(it was never about me, always about you)
I loved you like a dog[7]

To the brothers who mistreated and betrayed him, Joseph said, "You intended to harm me, but God intended it for good to accomplish what is now being done, the saving of many lives" (Genesis 50:20).

🌸

TIP: Use your pain. Get it out. Turn sad into art. Don't let if fester or grow into a bitter tree. Paint it, make it a poem or a joke or a song. Someone else will see or hear it and understand, and your empathy will comfort them and validate your pain.

I HaTe BeInG BaLD

Charm is deceptive, and beauty is fleeting;
but a woman who fears the Lord is to be praised.

PROVERBS 31:30

I have to lean on that verse from Proverbs 31.

Also, still no wigs or scarves express my personality correctly. Gypsy fortune teller? No. Too purple, too pink, too rebellious, too hip, too perfectly coiffed Country Club lady. All no.

My Raggedy Ann wig feels the most like me. When I'm bald, I feel stern, mean, manly, murderous. When I wear my Raggedy Ann wig, I start to do this little dance—a wavy arm, wavy leg jig. I can't help it. Costumes are important in creating a character. I learned this in the drama department at Furman and Auburn and learned it again at *Saturday Night Live*. You can change your attitude by changing your costume!

I march out of the house as Raggedy Ann, and my cop husband doesn't bat an eye. He behaves most of the day like Robocop. He has his ruts, habits, hours of grooming, lineup of shoes and clothes on the bed. He makes the bed. He's military. He eats the same lineup of boiled eggs split in half and seasoned with Tabasco, oregano, rosemary; exactly five grapes; one tablespoon of peanut butter; one apple; and four Hershey's dark chocolate kisses every morning. His car is immaculate. I can feel him wincing when I sit next to him in the passenger seat with my makeup, cup of coffee, books, cell, gum, and Isaiah workbook spilling out on my lap. I ask him why my comedic Raggedy Ann appearance doesn't embarrass him.

"Opposites attract," he says, retaining his deadpan expression.

We leave for another doctor's visit. At Vandy our wait time for my blood work, vitals, doctor, and infusion is zero. My name is called immediately. I suspect someone doesn't want Raggedy Ann sitting in the lobby too long making a spectacle of herself or minimizing the seriousness of the atmosphere. So I'm let right in.

Dr. Rexer appreciates my attempt at levity. He smiles quickly, blushes as if on cue, and then gets right to business. Very serious. "Okay, let's examine you." He takes his stethoscope out. I sit on the white paper examining table, and he says, "Let's see if Raggedy Ann is alive."

I love that. That he played along with me.

I ask if I can take a picture with him. He looks reluctant and wants to know where the picture is going. I laugh. "Not Facebook!"

I am not happy about this cancer thing. But, I believe God works for my good (Romans 8:28), and the Bible is true, and this life is short even if you live to one hundred. I will try to make the best of the situation.

I have some cancer jokes. Hoping to perform them soon at Zanies.

People wonder how cancer has changed my life. Well, I'm retired, so I wake up late, watch TV all day, and take pills. Nothing's changed.

My best friend since I was twelve, Elizabeth, is driving sixteen hours this weekend to see me. I think she thinks I'm dying.[1]

I was standing in the shower thinking of all my little aches and pains, and I thought of Jesus and how He endured every physical and emotional pain that we do: the cross, whipping, thorns on head, spear in side, unable to breathe, pain in his hands and feet, the humiliation, being betrayed by a close friend, the rejection of the Father because our sin was on Him. Every pain. Every temptation.

When she arrived, Elizabeth and I picked up our conversation as if no time had passed since 1970, but instead of discussing cheerleading tryouts, Karen Carpenter, or the English exam, we were discussing our children's upcoming weddings and our grandchildren, cancer, and death.

I was with Liz in tenth grade, during PE, the day her father died. Someone from the office came out on the field and said she was needed in the office. They said, "Vicki should come with her." We knew then it was something bad. Her healthy dad had died suddenly of a heart attack at age forty.

It was my first brush with death. I sat next to her on her bed in her room after the funeral. We didn't talk, just sat there. People were in the living room awkwardly shuffling around lots of casseroles.

I've always thought Liz was the classiest and most beautiful woman in the world. She's smart and artistic and humble, and she observes everything, and she really thinks about things.

She always sends me sunshine, and I always send her strawberries. We harmonize "Blowin' in the Wind" together every time we meet.

There is a friend that sticketh closer than a brother.

PROVERBS 18:24 KJV

An attractive friend said to me with a deadpan face, "Breast cancer? I had that. Takes about a year. Worst part—drainage tubes." Her matter-of-factness comforted me. I couldn't help it, but I stole a glance at her blouse. She looked good.

My friend Candy, who went through same cancer, insisted on juicing. She was adamant that I not blend but juice. What's the difference? She told me that she immersed herself in juiced carrots three times a day during chemo and never missed a day of work at her teaching job.

I asked Dr. Rexer about vitamins. "Don't eat a vitamin of broccoli. Eat the broccoli!"

God invented the broccoli, and it works best just the way it is, probably organic without the chemicals on it.

The only bad thing I can't quite stop are See's Lollypops at the end of a long, hard day.

I could never quit a habit. I have an addictive personality. If I found comfort in something, I had to repeat it daily. The only way I could stop an addiction was to replace it with another addiction. Thus, the lollipops. Seems like the lesser of two evils. The apostle Paul famously said:

> For what I am doing, I do not understand. For what I will to do, that I do not practice; but what I hate, that I do. If, then, I do what I will not to do, I agree with the law that it is good. But now, it is no longer I who do it, but sin that dwells in me. For I know that in me (that is, in my flesh) nothing good dwells; for to will is present with me, but how to perform what is good I do not find. For the good that I will to do, I do not do; but the evil I will not to do, that I practice. Now if I do what I will not to do, it is no longer I who do it, but sin that dwells in me. I find then a law, that evil is present with me, the one who wills to do good. For I delight in the law of God according to the inward man. But I see another law in my members, warring against the law of my mind, and bringing me into captivity to the law of sin which is in my members. O wretched man that I am! Who will deliver me from this body of death? I thank God—through Jesus Christ our Lord! So then, with the mind I myself serve the law of God, but with the flesh the law of sin. (Romans 7:15–25 NLT)

At the risk of sounding like a confessional, but to hopefully endear myself to you with my naked honesty, I'll give you some shameful examples of my addiction. Bulimia in my gymnast days was replaced with constant bubble gum chewing and caffeine, then wine and cigarettes, which was then replaced with Diet Coke, wine, and some eating disorders, which were replaced with Coffee Nips, Diet Coke, and sunflower seeds, then See's Lollypops and Kangen Water. You get the picture. At least the habits are moving upward and healthier. Too old to be bad.

I was burdened with an oral fixation and finding comfort in food, gum, drink, and nail biting instead of God. I prayed and prayed for release. I could never just eat healthy because of my childhood issues.

Dad used to explain why he didn't say grace before meals. "I don't thank God for food, because we eat too much," he said. "Food is a curse, not a blessing."

That is a lie from the enemy. Food is a blessing from God.

I think we spend our first fifty years trying to undo the damage our parents did to us.

Maybe God used cancer to release me from this generational curse.

When I was five, my dad, who was my PE teacher and gymnastics coach, looked at my little puff of a tummy in my sweaty red leotard and said, "You should lose five pounds. You're okay for a normal person, but not for a gymnast." He then picked up a hot jumbo cashew from his steaming paper bag and in slow motion placed it into his mouth. Chewing, he continued, "Nuts are high in calories. It's a carbohydrate. We're carboholics. If I'd ever had a drink, I'd be an alcoholic, because the chemical makeup of alcohol and carbohydrates is very similar. But, I've never had a drink."

My mouth was drooling for a cashew. He finally gave me one. I savored every molecule of it. This was the beginning of my love-hate relationship with food. I feel guilty with every swallow.

I found my ten-year-old diary while cleaning the garage. The diary shows I was busy with church, gymnastics, ballet, movies, and friends. One entry says: *I'm saved, have been since seven years old and sometimes I feel maybe I'm not, but I know I am because I love Jesus with all my heart, and I try to act like a Christian.* Another entry says: *Today was the big meet at Fort Myers. We had to get up at 5:30 a.m. and leave the house at 6 a.m. I didn't win anything. Daddy says I'm too fat to do gymnastics. So I'm going on a diet.*

That about sums up my life. Performing, which is like being naked in public, then being critiqued—*You're fat.*

❧

New joke for my act:

My first thought when I heard cancer was suicide. But, I don't like guns or knives or pills. So, I thought, I know, I'll go to Martin Luther King Boulevard and shout "All lives matter!" No, I'll fly to Syria and go to an ISIS stronghold wearing an "I heart Jesus" T-shirt! No, I'll go to a mosque wearing a bikini and sing, "I am woman, hear me roar!"

I've been thinking about suicide. Dr. Rexer said, "Yes, you can have a recurrence of cancer, but it isn't always cancer that kills you, there are other things you can die from, like a car accident. He said one of his patients didn't show up for her checkup. He googled her and found out she had just died in a head-on collision.

(I suspect it could have been an on-purpose car accident.)

There's a new cocktail, I saw on *Oprah*, where if your suffering is unbearable, you just plan a time and place, write notes to your loved ones, or be hanging out with them, and then drink the concoction and go to sleep forever. This grieving husband told Oprah that it's not suicide because his dying wife did not choose to get inoperable brain cancer. She simply chose a more dignified way to leave.

If I have to get chemo again in a year or a couple years, after all this poison and radiation that is to come, I would contemplate suicide at least for a moment; instead of a slow, agonizing death that your sweet family watches sadly and helplessly, drink a little cocktail with an umbrella in it and go to sleep.

But then, there's God.

He breathes meaning into every moment. He has a plan. He is God, the one who decides when life begins and ends. When I told my friend Paula that suicide had whisked across my mind, she adamantly scolded, "No! What if there is one more person who you could have reached for Christ but you took your life the day before? He is using you now. Don't thwart His purposes!"

I remember the fear and struggle of being twenty years old. Old age isn't the only difficult age. I was living in Los Angeles with no family to lean on. I should have joined a church. They would have protected me, but I was distracted with thoughts of survival and trusting myself instead of God.

What will I eat today? I need a job. Oh yeah, I have three. Will my clunker car start? So I can get to my jobs. Are my checks bouncing?

One time I walked home from Hollywood Presbyterian because I had no car and a weirdo stranger followed me home to my rented hovel where I had no roommates. It scared me, so I didn't go back. One time, a stranger stuck his hand up my skirt in broad daylight on the street, once a man in a raincoat flashed me, and once I was held up by a man with a gun. I got away.

In my twenties, I was bursting with stuff to say. I went to Hollywood and got on stages, any stage, anywhere—bars, comedy clubs, American Cancer Society telethons. Anywhere people would look at me and listen to me. Strangers were like, "Okay, say it. Go ahead," just because I looked so desperate to be heard. Directors hired me. They could tell I would just explode if I didn't get to emote, exhale, be seen and heard!

Why did I have so much to emote?

For one thing, I had twenty-five years of Bible training brewing inside. I was taught since birth that my mission was to tell the gospel of Jesus Christ to the world, by whatever means possible. The eternal security of everyone was at stake. I took this seriously.

Then, I had eighteen years of gymnastically trained muscles and hormones bursting with enthusiasm and vigor, desperate to be used for something, anything. Emotionally I was dying to vent about my battle with puberty, whatever that mysterious thing was, and my discovery of dangerous sex and vodka, pot and musicians. Help!

And I think I just desperately wanted a hug. Living alone in shabby apartments, having no money, sharing a bathroom with five welfare recipients in my shanty five days a week, and then washing my hands in the gold-and-marble sink of the Playboy Mansion on weekends and being the only Baptist virgin there, and listening to Barbie Benton explain how she could tell real diamonds from cubic zirconia at the table where James Caan the movie star sat. Riding home at midnight on my moped past the dark office buildings and into the illegal alien neighborhood where I lived, hoping to slip into my one rented room before the murderers/rapists saw me. All of these stories were bursting to come out of me and be heard by someone.

But now, I look around and everything is old. Even my dog. Everything has been said a thousand times by others and said way better. "I think that I shall never see / A poem as lovely as a tree."[2] I can add nothing to that. "If you can keep your head when all about you / Are losing theirs and blaming it on you, / If you can trust yourself when all men doubt you, / But make allowance for their doubting too.[3] Can't say that better. None of my thoughts are original or new or young and brave. I'm world weary.

I vaguely remember when the world was young—everything was blooming and bursting with excitement and possibility.

Now, everything is limited to a small space. Reachable goals. One day I planted four little trees. That was a big thing. I used to fly to Los Angeles for a three-line audition! Now, I'm grateful if I don't have to drive to the grocery store and don't have vertigo, a cough, or nausea.

I taught my kids long ago when they were little: "Women are evil, men are pigs, and life sucks. But God is good." I'm surprised at just how true that little saying keeps proving itself. A friend from Husband's ex-cop world and his young voluptuous, barely-dressed wife just came to visit from Florida and were to have dinner with Husband. I had never heard of the couple before. Apparently, Husband had flown them in his chopper millions of times but had never introduced us or invited me to join them. I invited myself to this dinner. No one invited me. Her hoochi-mama blouse kept accidentally slipping off in the front every time Husband glanced in her direction. He then invited her to his men-only cigar club to hang out. The place I was never allowed. My stomach hurt so much that when I got home, I started looking for that Ativan that was stuffed under my bed somewhere with all those other cancer pill bottles.

Husband's favorite saying is, "Relationships are difficult." His other favorite saying is, "Sin always leads to heartache." I hope he remembers the second one every time a hoochi mama's blouse accidentally slips off in front of his face.

"Thou wilt keep him in perfect peace, whose mind is stayed on thee" (Isaiah 26:3 KJV).

TIP: Don't obsess on what others do to you or don't do to you. Obsess on Jesus.

HOT PINK WIGS

Wives, submit to your own husbands,
as to the Lord.

EPHESIANS 5:22–25

One day I got a text from a Tea Party acquaintance, who asked me if I'd looked into chlorine yet. Here's what the Internet said about it: "Chlorine belongs to the same chemical group as fluoride and belongs to a group of chemicals called pathogens."[1]

According to the Environmental Protection Agency, Americans are consuming 300–600 times the amount of chlorine that is considered safe to ingest. Chlorine is known as a persistent chemical, which means that unlike other sanitation chemicals, it does not break down.

The Environmental Defense Fund states that: "Although concentrations of these carcinogens (THMs) are low, it is precisely these low levels that cancer scientists believe are responsible for the majority of human cancers in the United States."[2]

Dr. Joseph M. Price said, "Chlorine is the greatest crippler and killer of modern times. It is an insidious poison."[3]

The US Council of Environmental Quality said, "Cancer risk among people drinking chlorinated water is 93 percent higher than among those whose water does not contain chlorine."[4]

So, I'm to never drink a glass of tap water or wine again, or of course smoke, no red lipstick (red dye is a carcinogen), never eat sugar, drink water from plastic bottles (only filtered water), not eat salmon from Outback because it is fed hormones (only eat wild salmon), only shop at Whole Foods and buy organic, no fast food, no smart meter on the house, don't put cell phone near my ear or in my bra, no blonde hair dye, and no microwave popcorn or microwave anything. And, no showers until I buy a chlorine blocker. Whew!

Cancer was a lot easier when Husband was being nice to me. We had a big disagreement about that voluptuous friend I'd never met before and about money last week, and he gave me the silent treatment for four days and nights. I know you're getting tired of this merry-go-round. Me too.

New jokes for my act:

We get along good when we're living in different states. When we're in the same state Husband says the same three things to me every day:

1. I picked up dog poop. (He resents my dog.)

2. I found a tick. (He squishes it in front of me.)

3. Where'd all the money go?

When I'm in a different state (I take my dog with me), we talk on the phone and Husband says a slightly different mantra every day:

1. Where'd all the money go?

2. I miss you.

Awww. Our last marriage therapist said, "The secret to staying married is to stay married."

I just found out what "Let's visit your parents in Florida really means." It's code for, "Let's go to Florida, so you can help your mom change your dad's diaper while I go to a bar at the beach with my cop buddies and watch bikinis walk by."

I've noticed women are nicer to me now. They treat me like I'm out of the competition, out of the beauty contest we entered in first grade, when everyone realized the girls outnumbered the boys so you'd have to compete to win one. Now that I'm a minus seven, I'm out of the pageant, in the bleachers. And men, young and old, when they hear my cancer news, get a soft, caring look in their eyes, like they are sad for me that I have no breasts and that they were savagely, torn, ripped, and cut off with a bloody knife. Also, they look sad, like their favorite potential toy on me is smashed.

I have a fantasy that when Husband leaves me, which by his recent behavior seems soon, I will find a man whose privates were also cut off, and he'll be attracted to me, and me to him, knowing that as Ben Carson, famous brain surgeon and presidential candidate, so eloquently said at the National Religious Broadcaster's Convention, 2015, "Sex is all in the brain." I was there. He really said that. It's true.

God made our bodies to reproduce. And to have babies. And to breastfeed. Some women's cancers are caused in their women parts from lack of usage. Some cancers are caused from multiple sex partners. We have to follow God's rules if we want maximum health and wellness. God created sex and reproduction pure and beautiful. We should enjoy it and celebrate it, within His boundaries.

Here are some verses about it: "Flee fornication" (1 Corinthians 6:18 KJV); "Thou shalt not commit adultery" (Exodus 20:14 KJV); "Children are a heritage from the Lord, an offspring, a reward from him. Like arrows in the hands of a warrior are children born in one's youth. Blessed is the man whose quiver is full of them" (Psalm 127:3–5); and "Your wife will be like a fruitful vine within your house; your children will be like olive shoots around your table" (Psalm 128:3).

I just learned the coolest thing from a Perry Stone video at my small group studying Revelation. Jewish customs are important in understanding Jesus' parables and metaphors. Many prophecies of Jesus as Messiah are seen in the foreshadowing rituals of Judaism, the Passover, the spotless lamb sacrifices, Abraham and Isaac, and more.

There are also many allusions in the Bible to the church (believers) being the bride of Christ, but no one had ever explained to me what the Jewish wedding customs entailed. When I learned it, all the verses I'd memorized my whole life lit up with deeper meaning.

First, the Jewish groom seeks out a woman. Jesus seeks us out ("He came to seek and to save the lost" [Luke 19:10 ESV]). He calls us out of darkness (1 Peter 2:9).

Next, the woman responds ("as many as received Him" [John 1:12]). She accepts conversation and then accepts dinner with the groom's father. The father, if he approves, offers a contract ("The Father, who has given them to me" [John 10:20]). The Bible is our contract. It is God's Word. The contract says the bridegroom will protect us, take care of us, even die for us (John 3:16), and we will obey Him and love Him with all our heart, soul, and mind ("And you must love the LORD your God with all your heart, all your soul, all your mind, and all your strength" [Mark 12:30 NLT]).

Then, the groom offers jewels to the bride. She accepts them. Jesus offers us promises of eternal life with Him in heaven where the streets are gold and there are jewels and mansions:

> The foundation stones of the city wall were adorned with every kind of precious stone [jasper, sapphire, chalcedony, emerald, sardonyx, sardius, chrysolite, beryl, topaz; the tenth, chrysoprase, jacinth, amethyst] … And the twelve gates were twelve pearls; each one of the gates was a single pearl. And the street of the city was pure gold, like transparent glass. I saw no temple in it, for the Lord God the Almighty and the Lamb are its temple. And the city has no need of the sun or of the moon to shine on it, for the glory of God has illumined it, and its lamp is the Lamb (Revelation 21:19–23 NASB).

The Jewish groom goes off with his father to their home country or town (the ascension, Luke 24), and the groom builds a room on to the family homestead for his bride ("In My Father's house are many dwelling places; if it were not so, I would have told you; for I go to prepare a place for you. If I go and prepare a place for you, I will come again and receive you to Myself, that where I am, there you may be also. And you know the way where I am going" [John 14:1–4 NASB]). The groom builds his bride's mansion with his father's help. It may take a year.

Tradition is that the bride then covers herself more modestly to show the town she is betrothed, engaged. Like an engagement ring. Jewish tradition then has the groom returning as a surprise ("The day of the Lord will come like a thief in the night" [1 Thessalonians 5:2]).

Maybe it's to keep his bride true and faithful and/or keep her on her toes, but according to Jewish tradition, many times the groom surprised her in the middle of the night.

She is delighted. She is anxiously awaiting her groom every day that year or two. ("The victor's crown of righteousness is now waiting for me, which the Lord, the righteous Judge, will give to me on the day that he comes, and not only to me but also to all who eagerly wait for his appearing" [2 Timothy 4:8 ISV]).

His coming is a mystery ("But of that day and hour no one knows, not even the angels of heaven, but My Father only" [Matthew 24:36 NKJV]). Jewish tradition says that only the groom and his father know the day he journeys back to gather his wife.

I'd always wondered about those verses. Now it all makes sense. It's a parallel to the traditional Jewish wedding. Jesus was Jewish. He was talking to Jews.

It's about the intimate relationship God wants to have with us. Love.

After fifty-six years of Bible study, I keep learning new things. This Bible, God's Word, is alive. It speaks to you where you are. God speaks to you individually. It was written by men who were divinely inspired by God (2 Timothy 3:16). And it is forbidden to add or subtract one "jot or tittle" (Matthew 5:18; see also Deuteronomy 4:2, Revelation 22:18). That refers to the tiniest marking in the written Hebrew alphabet.

I am not a good artist, but I doodled a picture to express my recent thoughts about going through the valley of the shadow of death. I kept reading that God would hold me with His righteous right hand (Isaiah 41:10). What is the significance of the right hand? Well, I realized the Bible often says that Jesus sits at the right hand of the Father. So, I was thinking that right hand may mean Jesus. God's right-hand man will hold us, pull us up when we fall, and guide us along earth's rocky journey. Because God is a spirit and cannot be seen, Jesus is the personification of God.

The picture came into my head. I drew a bald cancer patient lying in bed in the middle of the night, pondering life, death, and cancer, and God/Jesus, Father/Groom coming to comfort her with His touch, His promises, and His words of life. The big hand is Jesus, and His right hand is helping me.

I went to a friend's fiftieth birthday and saw some friends I hadn't seen in a year. I felt the need to explain my wig of purple/gray braids.

The reaction on people's faces when I tell them I have cancer usually follows this cycle: truly horrified, pity, sympathy, don't want to catch it, visualize me dying soon and how it will affect their lives, culminating in encouragement to stay strong. They are sincere and caring. What I usually say back is: "I've been through worse things."

When I asked Dr. Rexer if I could take the seven hundred dollars' worth of supplements my brother James sent me, to heal me, Dr. Rexer recommended the book, *In Defense of Food*, and said, "I prefer a glass of red wine, salmon, and a whole-wheat roll. My wife bakes homemade bread." He looked up dreamily like he couldn't wait to get home and away from all these diseased middle-aged women.

Husband interjected jealously, "She bakes homemade bread!"

Dr. Rexer said, "She has a PhD in cancer research, we met in med school, but she gave it up to raise our four children."

Husband said, "A PhD and homemade bread!"

I couldn't help but feel a stab of disdain from Hubbie. *Hmph*! I bet she never did a handstand on the Update Desk!

Dr. Rexer nodded proudly and continued, "For seven hundred dollars, you could eat foie gras duck flown in from—"

"But, my brother already paid for these. Can I take them when chemo is over, so they aren't wasted?"

Dr. Rexer thinks antioxidants might mess up the effects of chemo.

"Sure, they won't hurt you after chemo is done."

On the TV in my chemo room, I see a young Johnny Crawford in The Rifleman. *I've known him since 1980 when he discovered me in Birmingham summer stock. He was the star from Hollywood flown in for* Meet Me in St. Louis, *and I was the chorus line girl doing back handsprings. He thought I had a funny voice and a thirties personality. I did a handstand on a chair and a fire hydrant to get his attention. He gave me a one-way ticket to Hollywood to be in his thirties night club act. I'd never seen the TV show he was famous for until chemo! I took a selfie and sent it to him.*[5]

I remember meeting his costar, Chuck Connors, in Beverly Hills after Johnny took me to the Emmys. I was wearing a sheer vintage green gown from a thrift shop and was very thin and young. I hadn't been on any TV shows yet and found the Emmys pretty boring in general. But, I felt pretty in my tattered green gown. Chuck Connors was old, maybe sixty-five. I was twenty. He asked me if I wanted to have sex with him! We had just met! I told him I was a Baptist virgin. He looked at Johnny to see if this was a joke! Johnny nodded no, and smiled whimsically, like it's not a joke. Me and Johnny drove off in his 1929 Chrysler.

I thought about the first time Johnny had driven me to the Playboy Mansion in his 1929 Chrysler. Johnny sang 1930s classics, like "There's a Tear for Every Smile in Hollywood" (written by Sam Stept and Bud Green). His heart lives in that era, as mine does. I was born at the wrong time. I remember asking Johnny why he would never take me to the mansion where he went every weekend while I stayed in my tiny room at the Kipling Retirement Hotel where I worked for room and board, after my American Cancer Society typing job.

"I'll never find an agent if I can't go anywhere to meet anyone."

Johnny replied, "I don't want you to change."

"What do you mean?"

"All the girls who go to the Playboy Mansion start drinking and smoking and get breast implants."

"Oh. I won't change."

Johnny drove me up to the big, famous gates, where he told a big rock with a speaker in it his famous name and the name of his guest, me.

We entered the castle, I in my thrift shop ensemble (cuffed shorts, a purple bow tie, white shirt, and red high heels). I met Hef, a lot of perfect-looking Playboy girls, old comics, Shannon Tweed, and Shel Silverstein, the poet who wore a baggy long beige muumuu. I did some handstands in the backyard and Johnny took a picture. I swam in the pool in a borrowed bikini from the bikini bin and felt wild and crazy for a minute. I saw the grotto, but no one was having sex or doing drugs anywhere that I could see.

I glance away from *The Rifleman* TV show and snap back to reality. Poison is dripping into my veins from a bag hanging on a pole. I have cancer. I am on the verge of divorce number two.

I think, *Hey, Vanderbilt and The Playboy Mansion have a lot in common—all breasts all the time.*

After chemo, I go alone to the Sally Field movie *Hello, My Name is Doris* and realize I'd read the script somewhere! Had I turned it down? Sally Field is wearing my hairdo! She has her hair piled on top of her head with a big bow stuck in there in every scene! Had the writer/director told her to look like me? It is a quirky, funny movie until the end when the twenty-five-year-old guy that seventy-year-old Sally/Doris has a crush on decides to date her despite their age difference, and he kisses her on the mouth. Ew! That's probably why I turned it down. But, I should have taken it! It's not a sin to date someone that much younger, is it? Well, it seems wrong. I can't think of a Bible verse about it though.

I then go to a different movie theater alone and see *Climate Hustle*, a documentary proving that global warming and climate change is a hoax created to control the masses and redistribute the wealth. I knew that already, but the movie did a great job at proving it. I must bribe my kids into seeing this. They need to know the truth.

I am killing time because I want Husband to worry about me, and have a little taste of what it would be like to be divorced from me. He'd be lonely! I'm fun, right?

So, then I visit Mom. And then, I come home.

Husband is on the porch smoking a cigar. He said he was worried about me and was on the verge of calling the police. "I didn't know where you were."

"Well," I replied, "when we're divorced, you'll never know where I am," and I waltzed in the house.

My plan worked.

Later that night, Paul reminded me that we'd RSVP'd to the Franklin Graham thing, "Decision America." I can't miss that.

We both drive together to the event at 9:00 a.m. I use the opportunity of Husband being trapped with me in a car to give him a thirty-minute monologue on the inappropriateness and cruelty of him telling my flaws to Aubrey's college professor for her "interview the parents" project.

Husband and I attend the Franklin Graham event, and our hearts melt at the beauty of Jesus, his love, his gospel, and his people. A sweet spirit permeates the air as thousands of Jesus followers fill the Legislative Plaza in front of the Capitol to pray for our country and for forgiveness.

Franklin Graham is humble and witty and warm. He says, "Daddy is ninety-seven years old. He thinks nobody remembers him."

The crowd laughs loud.

"Daddy said, 'Well, if anyone remembers me, tell them I said hi.'"

The crowd laughs again.

Franklin reads the story of Nehemiah leading Israel to repent before God. And like Nehemiah, we ask God to forgive our country for disobedience, abortion, and immorality. There is a soft mumble across the crowd as we list our nation's sins out loud. Next, he tells us to repent silently for our own sins. Then, like Nehemiah, he admonishes us to ask God for forgiveness for the sins of our fathers.

Franklin continues, "My dad is a good man, and my dad's dad was a good man, but we have some bad men in our family tree. I know some of you had a bad man for a father."

Charlie Daniels sings, "I'll Fly Away," and Michael W. Smith leads us in "Amazing Grace." Franklin encourages us to vote for candidates with biblical values and run for office ourselves. I tell Husband again that he would be a great candidate.

I bump into a friend of Chonda Pierce walking to the parking lot, and I tell her I have cancer. She prays for me right there on the street.

Husband holds my hand, and when no one is watching kisses me on the mouth.

I think he's trying to win me back.

Dr. Rexer looks pretty surprised at my next visit when we ask him if I'm allowed to have sex during chemotherapy.

"Use Me"

The Actress cries out from her lonely apartment
"Use me, Use me"

The Abandoned Wife in her curlers and nightgown cries
"Use me, please use me."
The Man in the Sombrero Hat at the Bar, he says,
"Use me. C'mon. Use This!"
Silently everyone desperately wants to be used.

Isn't if funny just how we were made
When we are used, we feel jaded
When we are needed, we cry out for help,
"Leave me alone. I'm not at home.
I won't answer my phone."
Isn't it funny how everyone thinks they're being used?[6]

Mom and Dad's cemetery plot salesman keeps calling me. He knows I have cancer because I wore a wig to Dad's crypt ceremony. Six months ago, I was holding a handstand for a preschool commercial and performing live at Zanies, and now I'm the target of a cemetery plot salesman who is excited that I have cancer and am dying soon, so he can make a sale!

This death thing is getting too close. I liked it better when it was a faraway concept we sang about in church.

Remembering Dad, I'm thinking, *Maybe it's better to die at fifty-six instead of eighty-seven.*

Proverbs 17:22 says, "A cheerful heart is good medicine, but a crushed spirit dries up the bones."

TIP: When you're preparing to make love to your husband, don't put your hot, itchy hot-pink wig on until you hear your husband coming up the stairs. If you put it on three hours before you hear footsteps, the sweat will make your sexy makeup drip off.

To see see these pictures in color, please visit VictoriaJackson.com.

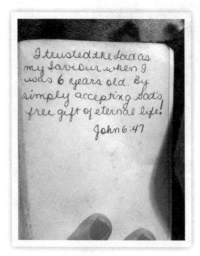

I trusted the Lord as my Saviour when I was 6 years old. By simply accepting God's free gift of eternal life!
John 6:47

My childhood Bible.

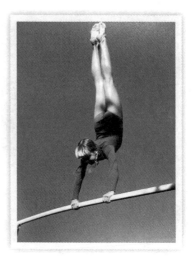

My backyard, 1970.

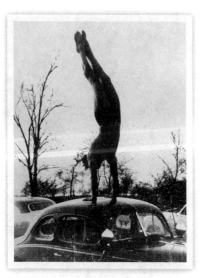

My dad on his 1949 Ford Opera Coupe.

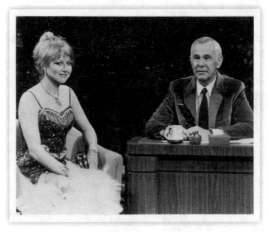

The Tonight Show starring Johnny Carson, 1983.

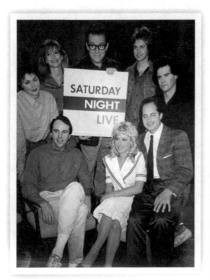

SNL cast, 1986–1992.

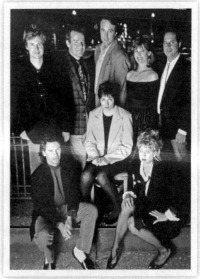

SNL cast, 1986–1992.

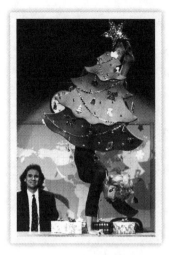

SNL Update Desk, 1989.
(photo by Sissi Stein-Schneider)

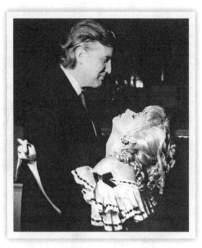

Me and Donald Trump, photo shoot for
People magazine, 1992.

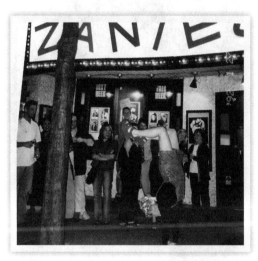

Zanies Comedy Club, Chicago, 2002.

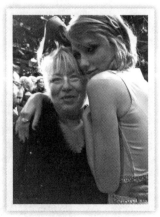

Me and Taylor Swift,
SNL 40th Reunion, 2015.

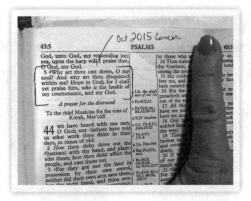

The verse God gave me after I was diagnosed with cancer.

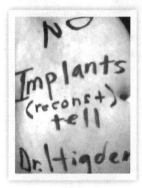

Instructions to the doctors
before surgery.
Yes, that's my stomach.

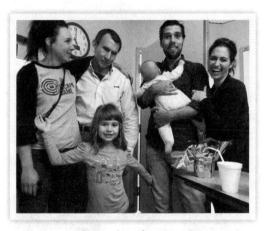

When I woke up from surgery.

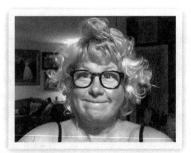

Still have hair after first chemo.

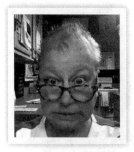

Baldish after second chemo.

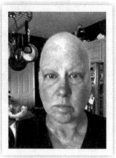

Bald – I look like
Christopher Hitchens.

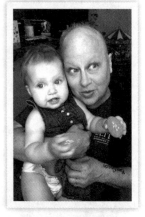

Me and my grandbaby.

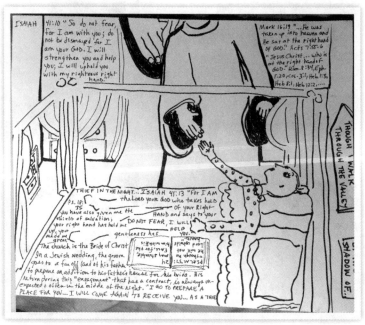

My doodlings during chemo.

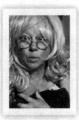

Perky blonde.

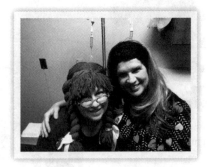

Raggedy Ann with nurse Christine.

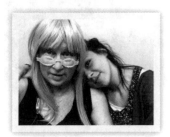

My lavender gray wig with
daughter Aubrey.

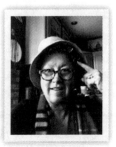

Hat on loan from
friend Candy.

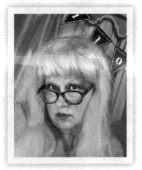

Hot pink.

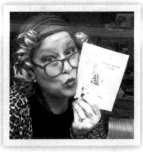

My expensive curly blonde wig.

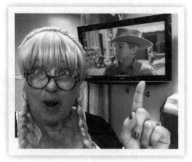

Johnny Crawford on *The Rifleman*.

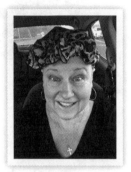

Leopard scarf gift
from Debi.

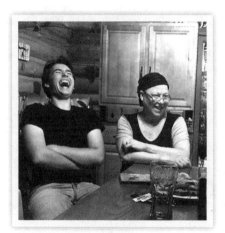

Jacob Dufour (star/screenwriter of
Andy's Rainbow) and me.

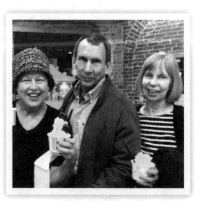

Best friends since 1970—me, Paul, Elizabeth.

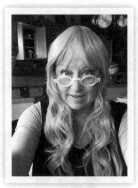

Long pink wig.

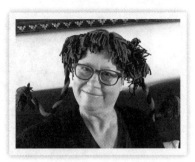

Pippi Longstocking.

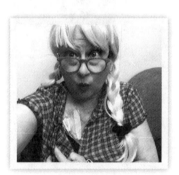

My port.

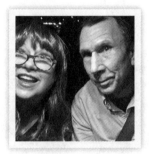

On a date.

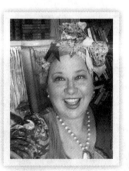

My most creative head
covering endeavor.

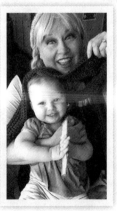

Handmade purple scarf
from dear Glenn.

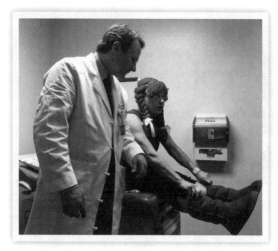

My checkup.

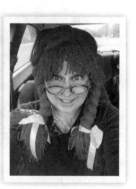

Raggedy Victoria.

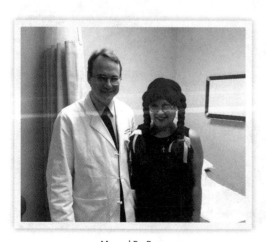

Me and Dr. Rexer.

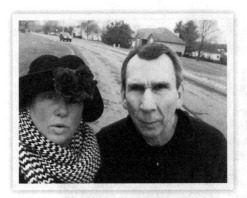

Romantic winter walk.

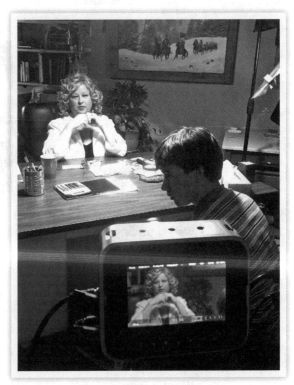

Filming *Andy's Rainbow*, 2016.

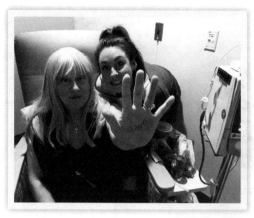

With Aubrey.

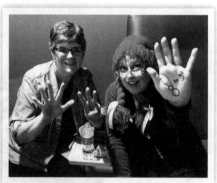

With Patty.

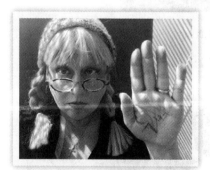

Seven chemo treatments to go.

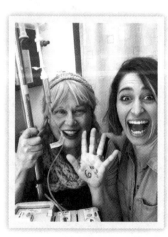

With Scarlet.

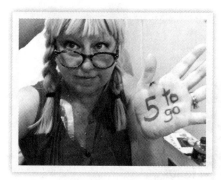

Five chemo treatments to go.

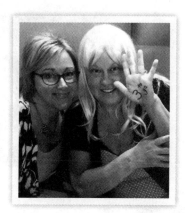

With Judy.

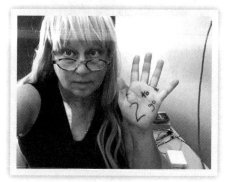

Two chemo treatments to go.

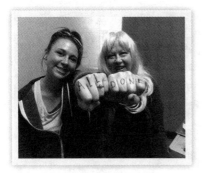

With Aubrey.

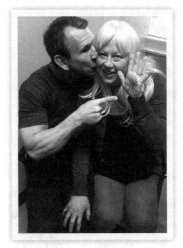

With Paul.

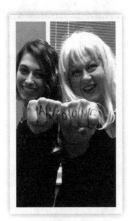

With Scarlet.

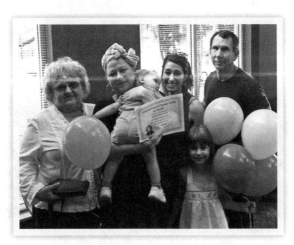

My thirty-third and last radiation.

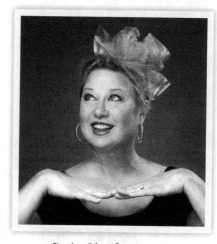

First headshot after treatment
(photo by Dieter Spears).

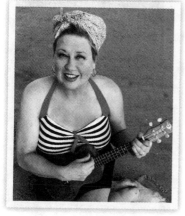

Platinum Planet song-writing camp
at Oak Island, NC, post-treatment.

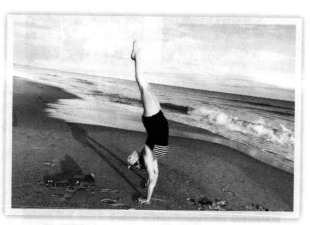

You can do a handstand even after cancer!

A Serious Role

All Scripture is God-breathed and is useful for teaching,
rebuking, correcting and training in righteousness.

2 Timothy 3:16

*A*t my next appointment, I made three lab-coated doctors laugh all at once. Dr. Rexer and two observers walked into my examining room. There wasn't much to talk about. Doc said my blood numbers are excellent. I told him that I have no side effects. One brief nerve tingling in the hands. Then, I asked him if I could do this movie, *Andy's Rainbow*, I was just offered in Indiana, playing the role of a doctor in a white coat.

The room erupted in laughter!

"My character is completely normal, not ditzy, not funny." I continued, "She runs a mental institution."

Gales of laughter ensued.

I laughed. "I could win an Oscar!"

The room was laughing so hard that Dr. Rexer pushed the wrong button on the computer and released me from chemo.

When I got to my chemo room with the IV drip bag of poison, there was no poison and my nurse, Christine, looking at the computer said, "Dr. Rexer ended your chemo? Didn't you have two left?"

That's what the Sharpie number on my hand said!

She made some calls. It was an error. More poison required. I guess I really did make them laugh!

❀

One night I ate ten See's Lollypops in a row. I got weary of my strict regimen. I guess my default face is lollipop mouth. Life seems not worth living without sugar!

I believe the cure to cancer is right under our noses. It's probably something really simple. Like no sugar.

Maybe the person who was going to discover cancer's cure was one of the fifty million babies murdered in America by abortion.

I was at the Democratic National Convention in 2012 when the Democrat Party voted God out of their platform. I was there as a journalist for Liberty Alliance. Pro-abortion activists lined the streets shouting, "It's my body!" I was thinking, *But your DNA is different than the DNA of the human in your stomach.* One brave man protesting the Democrat Party platform held a large ten-foot-square photo of an aborted baby. No one could look at it.

They can do it but not look at it.

I asked my dad once, "Why doesn't Jesus just come back already?" Dad pointed to 2 Peter 3:9: "The Lord is not slack concerning His promise … but is longsuffering toward us, not willing that any should perish but that all should come to repentance" (NKJV). Maybe God is waiting for that one more person to come to Him. Reader, it might be you.

I'm looking out the window at the snow one day, eating my homemade soup made of organic kale, carrots, celery, peppers, onions, cheese, squash, beans, turkey, Brussel sprouts, radishes, broccoli, garlic, turmeric, rosemary, basil, and pepper. I just finished my eight-fruit-and-veggie smoothie. I decide to google turmeric. I've turned into a health nut. An article I find on the Internet lists these warnings and precautions:

> Hormone-sensitive condition such as breast cancer, uterine cancer, ovarian cancer, endometriosis, or uterine fibroids: Turmeric contains a chemical called curcumin, which might act

like the hormone estrogen. In theory, turmeric might make hormone-sensitive conditions worse. However, some research shows that turmeric reduces the effects of estrogen in some hormone-sensitive cancer cells. Therefore, turmeric might have beneficial effects on hormone-sensitive conditions. Until more is known, use cautiously if you have a condition that might be made worse by exposure to hormones.[1]

Uh oh. My cancer feeds on estrogen, and turmeric acts like estrogen, but sometimes turmeric reduces the effects of estrogen in some hormone-sensitive cancer cells. Now, what am I supposed to do? Science don't know nothing.

I ask Dr. Rexer.

He says, "Use it as a spice. Sprinkle it. Not Costco size."

At one point, a friend from Florida and I reunited on the phone. We both got diagnosed with breast cancer the same year. We compared notes, thinking the cause of our cancer was marital stress. We've both quit sugar (well, I did have some bubble gum and one lollipop last night … and six Coffee Nips). They gave her six weeks to live, and she's still alive eighteen months later.

M. never drank or smoked.

Science has made great advances but is still in the dark about cancer. They are experimenting on us.

Two years ago, I was driving through the local Starbucks for my Venti Caffè Frappuccino with coconut milk, only three pumps of the base, and an added shot of decaf, when Joshua, the cute guy with the blonde beard and the tattoos *LOVE* and *HOPE* on his arms, leaned out the window and said, "Can I pray with you? Oh, and I have a word from the Lord for you."

I was happily startled. This must be the Bible Belt. Where else do you get a prayer at the drive-through?

Joshua said, "One, you have been faithful in your relationships. Two, your family is in a season of rest. Three, opportunities will come that were put on hold because of circumstances."

The weird thing is, he used almost the exact words I had just prayed the night before. I had written it down somewhere. I had told God that I just wished I could get a nod, a pat on the back or something, to know if I was doing the right thing with my life. Was I pleasing Him? The opportunities part I assumed meant the acting roles that had disappeared when I moved to Miami to raise a family with Husband. Soon after this word from Joshua, five movie roles fell into my lap. This was fulfilling for me.

The "season of rest" phrase stuck in my head. It was great news except that it carried a warning, that the season of rest was temporary, it was a season. Uh oh. I kept thinking, *God must be preparing me for something big, some challenge.*

The challenge must have meant cancer.

Driving with our five-year-old granddaughter Ever is always entertaining. She sings, improvising songs for whatever is happening at the moment, just like her dad and mom and Gran and me and my mom do. Husband is always in deadpan cop face. Our lives look and sound like a Disney musical but with a grumpy Indian chief in the middle of every scene. We were explaining to Ever why Bam Bam's (they call me Bam Bam) chest was suddenly flat and bandaged and her hair falling out. This is a transcript from our car conversation. It isn't perfect theology, just real life. I turned on my cell video and prodded her to talk about it.

Me: Okay, Ever, say that over again, so I can video it.

Ever: Okay, so I was saying that Bam Bam's sick-a-ness, it's a disease. It's where Jesus might fix you, um, um, while you're back on earth, or He might just, or you might just have it forever. We don't know.

Me: And so you said, "That's a little bit sad?"

Ever: Yeah. It is because it's sad if you don't get better.

Me: Right. And then you said, "I don't know why Jesus wouldn't heal you. 'Member you said that?"

Ever: Yeah. I don't know why He won't heal you, if He can do anything.

Me: That's right.

Ever: He has a plan to make her better.

Me: Who has a plan?

Ever: Jesus. I trust Him that He has a plan. He has a plan for us. He runs the world. He takes care of us. He knows what to do. He has a plan. He runs the world.

Me: You're right, Ever.

Ever: He has a plan to make her better.

Me: So what do you think is going to happen to Bam Bam and her disease?

Ever: I don't know. I don't know yet. Jesus hasn't told me. But, I'll see if He can tell me right now. (She bows her head.)

Me: Oh, you're so cute.

Ever: I know. I know what it is.

Me: Did He tell you? What did He say?

Ever: He told me (she looks out the window up to the stars in the night sky) up there, He told me that He, He's going to … He, He, He doesn't know yet, but He, He said, He's going to do something good, and He's just going to make you better … but He said, on earth, but we don't know what way it's going to happen, but …

Me: Right. He's going to do something good.

Ever: He's gonna do something good.

Me: Praise the Lord.

SCARLET: Tell us your Bible verse.

Ever: "The grass dies. The flower fades. But, God's Word stands
   forever!"

Me: Amen!

Ever: Turn that off! (referring to the camera)

I must remember to tell Ever that I won't have cancer forever
according to 1 Corinthians 15:

> It is the same way with the resurrection of the dead. Our earthly
> bodies are planted in the ground when we die, but they will
> be raised to live forever. Our bodies are buried in brokenness,
> but they will be raised in glory. They are buried in weakness,
> but they will be raised in strength. They are buried as natural
> human bodies, but they will be raised as spiritual bodies. For
> just as there are natural bodies, there are also spiritual bodies. …
>
> Adam, the first man, was made from the dust of the earth,
> while Christ, the second man, came from heaven. Earthly peo-
> ple are like the earthly man, and heavenly people are like the
> heavenly man. Just as we are now like the earthly man, we will
> someday be like the heavenly man.
>
> What I am saying, dear brothers and sisters, is that our
> physical bodies cannot inherit the kingdom of God. These
> dying bodies cannot inherit what will last forever.
>
> But let me reveal to you a wonderful secret. We will not all
> die, but we will all be transformed! It will happen in a moment,
> in the blink of an eye, when the last trumpet is blown. For when
> the trumpet sounds, those who have died will be raised to live
> forever. And we who are living will also be transformed. For
> our dying bodies must be transformed into bodies that will
> never die; our mortal bodies must be transformed into immor-
> tal bodies.

Then, when our dying bodies have been transformed into bodies that will never die, this Scripture will be fulfilled:

> "Death is swallowed up in victory.
> O death, where is your victory?
> O death, where is your sting?"

For sin is the sting that results in death, and the law gives sin its power. But thank God! He gives us victory over sin and death through our Lord Jesus Christ." (vv. 42–44, 47–57 NLT)

It sounds like little Ever Grace has had some Bible training. I can't help but compare her Bible teaching to the opposite indoctrination that leads Islamic mothers who send their seven-year-olds to jihadist training camps to learn to kill, as described in books like *The Blood of Lambs*. One child is being taught love. The other child is being taught hate.

Liberals equate Christianity with Islam and say that both religions have extremists. However, that statement is untrue on many levels. First of all, an extreme Muslim will kill you. An extreme Christian will love you to death! Christianity and Islam are opposite. Mohammed said, "Kill the infidel (the non-Muslim)." Jesus said, "Love your enemies, bless them that curse you" (Matthew 5:44 KJV).

Secondly, Christianity is not a religion. The root of the word religion is *religio*, which means "to bind back to God." Religion teaches good works for salvation. The Bible teaches in Ephesians 2:8–9, "For by grace you have been saved through faith; and that not of yourselves, it is a gift of God; not of works lest any man should boast" (NASB).

Christianity is a relationship, not a religion. It teaches that God died for us, so that we could live with Him eternally (John 3:16).

Islam is a works-for-salvation religion that teaches that you must die for Allah to gain eternal life. Islam is a military and political system, a theocracy. Sharia law controls every aspect of a Muslim's life, and there is no separation of church and state.

Our Constitution gives freedom of religion.

Islam's holy book, the Quran, was written 600 years after the Bible, using its stories and changing the names around.

The Bible was written by over forty authors who lived at different times over 2,000 years, and it has one message—the gospel.

The Quran was written by one man, Mohammed, who was violent and encouraged violence in his followers.

Jesus taught peace. Jesus rose from the grave.

Mohammed did not. No one even claimed Mohammed did.

Unbelievers, including the Jewish historian Josephus, reported on Jesus' resurrection.

Jesus never married and taught sexual purity and equality of the sexes.

Mohammed had many wives, married Aisha when she was six, consummated the marriage when she was nine, and endorsed polygamy and misogyny. He taught stoning as punishment for adultery.

Jesus stopped the stoning of the woman caught in adultery by saying, "He that is without sin among you, let him first cast a stone at her" (John 8:7 KJV).

Is the Muslim God Allah and the Jewish/Christian God Jehovah the same God? Absolutely not. They are opposite.

Jehovah, Yahweh, I AM, God says, "… that you may know that you have eternal life" (1 John 5:13).

Allah is unpredictable. There is no eternal security for a Muslim, and your best chance at heaven is being a suicide bomber.

But, I digress.[2]

God said in Proverbs 8:36, "All those who hate me love death" (NKJV).

I have set before you life and death, blessings and curses. Now choose life, so that you and your children may live.

Deuteronomy 30:19

Doesn't it all come down to life and death? Choose life.

I heard Hal Prince on TBN saying that the Bible is not ink on a page, but God's actual breath on every page. Second Timothy 3:16 says, "All Scripture is inspired by God." Another word for "inspired" is *breathed*. The Bible is God's breath, His Word speaking to us. The Word is Jesus.

"In the beginning was the Word and the Word was with God and the Word was God" (John 1:1).

TIP: Let God breathe on you every day, talk to you. Next, talk back to Him. Then, sit and listen. If that voice you hear lines up with Scripture, it's Him talking to you, not your conscience or your imagination. Husband and I read the Bible together every night and pray together, even in the bad times, especially in the bad times.

movie in indiana

Husbands, love your wives, just as Christ loved
the church and gave himself up for her.

EPHESIANS 5:25

I want to skip my last chemo. I always complete assignments.
However, the first day of my movie shoot is the day after my last
chemo, and I'll be at my weakest and puffiest. I call twice to try and
wiggle out of the last chemo, and two different nurses give me a pep
talk. They tell me I'm doing great and that other women in times past
were used as experiments to come up with this magical number of
treatments that I am now benefitting from. I finished the four doses
of the Red Devil combo, and now agree to the eleventh of twelve
Taxols. Sigh.

The only side effects now are fatigue, a mild tingling in my hands,
slight pain in big toe nails, and an overall creepy poisoned-to-death
feeling and baldness. I keep thinking that in a few years people will
laugh at this like we laugh at the stupidity of bloodletting (withdraw-
ing blood from a patient to cure or prevent illness, practiced from
1000 BC by the Egyptians, through the Greeks and Romans, and then
all the way up to the 1800s).

My curly blonde wig is the perfect wig for my new movie role as
Dr. Kennedy, the white-coated non-ditzy, caring professional head of
a mental institution. When I tell people my new role, they all burst
out in laughter.

I'm just happy to get away from a husband who doesn't love me.
Today I drew a cartoon expressing my pain. I have to get the pain out

somehow. His Florida cigar buddies are in town, so he's not going with me to Indiana. He's choosing them over me. He's choosing a week of bar hopping with the guys over a free hunting lodge get-away with a sick, bald wife. In my drawing, he's dancing on my bald head while he holds a cigar. I drive my sick self to Indiana alone.

This sets our marriage back decades. Maybe our marriage will never heal from this betrayal.

After chemo and before radiation, I got this two-week break, and God managed to give me a movie role to squeeze right into that time frame. Wow!

To radiate or not to radiate. That was the new question.

After the ten-day movie shoot, I am to begin six weeks of daily radiation. I push that thought aside to focus on my new movie role as Dr. Kennedy.

My arms have never been this flabby. My self-confidence has never been this low. I look in the mirror and say, "I am not an animal." I have weird poofs of fat at the end of my chest scars. These must be removed. Maybe when Dr. Grau surgically takes my port out, and I'm knocked out on that great drug, she can slice these globs off. I guess she left them there in case I was getting breast implants and they needed some skin to stretch across it. I don't know. I feel like a Dr. Frankenstein experiment. All glued together. A beat-up, bald-headed doll that some mean kid ripped the hair out of.

But, God.

God gave me a movie role during all of this. Isn't God amazing? He knew what my favorite thing in the whole world would be. And, I'm working with these amazing Christians in Indiana. There are wild-flowers, trees, and barns everywhere.

And, an eighteen-year-old home-schooled boy, Jacob Dufour, wrote the script. His mom is the craft service. His dad, a logger, who built the log cabin they live in, is producing/codirecting it with his son, who stars in the movie.

The mood is peaceful and joyful. Unlike Los Angeles and New York, no one is swearing. There are no egos. No demands. No tempers. No prima donnas. It's weird.

Jacob, the writer/director/actor, liked my suggestion to put my cancer into the movie. So, I take my wig off in one scene and show my bald head. This gives my character a backstory, more depth.

I play a doctor in a white coat who runs a mental hospital.

That sentence cracks me up. And, it's not a comedy!

It reminds me of my first Hollywood movie role—a nurse named Nurse Grabatit. They actually made a nametag for my uniform with that on it. I still have it somewhere. The movie was a comedy called *Stoogemania*. It was the story of a hospital where guys go who can't stop acting like the Three Stooges. My nurse character ended up doing a handstand on a table of food and then falling into the punch bowl.

I got meatier roles after that, working with big stars like Sean Connery, Dustin Hoffman, Diane Keaton, and Robert Downey Jr.

But, I digress.

They say chemo is cumulative, so you feel the worst on your last day. That's the day I drove myself to Indiana because Husband went to the City Winery and several other bars with his buddies. Yes, I'm mad. Hurt, really. Deeply wounded. But, I finished my last round of chemo! What a beautiful ring that has! *Last round.*

My friend Sue's husband celebrated her last round of chemo with a trip to Paris for the two of them. My husband celebrated without me by bar hopping with the Cigar Addicts (good name for a band) and his millionaire friend who owns the cigar company.

Murphy's Law says, "Anything that can go wrong, will go wrong." Some people add, "And usually at the worst time." The identity of Murphy is unknown, but the saying was first used during the 1940s and may have originated with members of the armed forces in World War II.

Well, I kinda told the director of this movie, *Andy's Rainbow*, that I had cancer *after* he gave me the role. Hey! It's hard to get acting roles!

It's almost impossible! That's why big movie stars are doing TV, and TV stars are now doing faith-based films. That's code for "Christian." I think cancer might be a plus though. My character is not the romantic lead. I don't have to be young, healthy, and beautiful. I could be a mess. And, messes are very interesting to watch on film.

However, I must be extra professional and not let my sickness be in any way a deterrent to the success of the shoot or the film. That's why I have to blame it on the devil or Murphy's Law that absolutely everything went wrong leading up to my big scenes.

My four-hour drive from Tennessee to Indiana turned into six because of a traffic jam, a GPS error, getting lost, and a flash flood. Husband chose to be with Cigar Magnate instead of his wife, so my heart was broken. My face is red and puffy. My eyes are slits. I get to the hunting lodge and find that my bathroom is down the hall. I am not allowed to put toilet paper in the toilet, there is no ice, the fan above my bed makes a loud, inconsistent banging noise (it's not white noise), I'm hot, and there are five dogs, two of which are barking at 6:00 a.m.

I couldn't sleep all night. I tried so hard. Because of rain, the schedule had been changed, and all of my lines, my big scenes, and close-ups were switched to Thursday.

Thursday was the day the chemo's effects would be peaking. You see, when I got chemo each Monday for the last five months, the steroids would stave off fatigue for a couple days, then Wednesday and especially Thursday, I'd feel the worst. The tingling hands, the painful toenails, the metal taste on the tongue, the fatigue. I'm grateful that I did not react as badly as some patients, but still, it's poison.

I bit the bullet. I prayed, *Lord, we want this movie to bring glory to you and souls into heaven, so please bless my performance and help me remember my lines despite my exhaustion.*

Donna, the script supervisor, prayed for me, and Adam, the director, started the day with prayer.

The night after all my close-ups, I slept twelve hours with the help of a white noise fan the director brought me, an air cleanser, and a bunch of juiced fruits and veggies from the director's wife. I woke up feeling fantastic. Of course, no close-ups of me that day.

There is a lilac bush outside my door here at the hunting lodge in Indiana where I'm staying to shoot the movie. Each time I pass it, the most exhilarating whiff fills my head and chest as if God is sprinkling blessings all over me, and into me, as I walk through the end of this valley of the shadow of death.

I was off today, so I poked around the little town of Salem and had a blast in the antique store. I found a cigar Indian for Husband's birthday and a big gold mirror from an estate sale, some rose china, a sparkling pink cat pin for one daughter, bookends with my grandkids' initials, and a Christmas deer antlers pin for Mom. God knows this is a heavenly day for me.[1]

Kevin Sorbo e-mailed and asked me for Jon Lovitz' e-mail. He had a role for him in a new movie. So, I texted Lovitz and got to catch up a little.

Ever since I sent Lovitz a Jewish tract (gospel literature) in his Christmas card, he brings up Jesus or being born again.

One time Jon and I were in Atlantic City, New Jersey, doing stand-up. It was me, Lovitz, and Kevin Nealon as the headliner. Jon and Kevin came over to my hotel room to hang out before the show. Husband and my kids were hanging out too.

After some chitchat, Jon says, "You can't be Jewish and Christian. That's like oil and vinegar. They don't mix!"

I said, "Jesus was Jewish! All the disciples were Jewish! Almost everyone in the Bible is Jewish!"

Lovitz continued, "How can a grown man crawl back into his mother's womb and be born again?"

I did a double take. "You're quoting Scripture!" I ran over to the drawer next to the bed where I'd seen a Gideon Bible. I didn't know that I knew exactly where the Nicodemus passage was, but I quickly turned right to John 3. I grabbed my video camera (this was before iPhones were invented) and asked Jon to read it aloud. He graciously complied. I videoed him reading:

There was a man of the Pharisees named Nicodemus, a ruler of the Jews. This man came to Jesus by night and said to Him, "Rabbi, we know that You are a teacher come from God; for no one can do these signs that You do unless God is with him."

Jesus answered and said to him, "Most assuredly, I say to you, unless one is born again, he cannot see the kingdom of God."

Nicodemus said to Him, "How can a man be born when he is old? Can he enter a second time into his mother's womb and be born?"

Jesus answered, "Most assuredly, I say to you, unless one is born of water and the Spirit, he cannot enter the kingdom of God. That which is born of the flesh is flesh, and that which is born of the Spirit is spirit. Do not marvel that I said to you, 'You must be born again.' The wind blows where it wishes, and you hear the sound of it, but cannot tell where it comes from and where it goes. So is everyone who is born of the Spirit."

Nicodemus answered and said to Him, "How can these things be?"

Jesus answered and said to him, "Are you the teacher of Israel, and do not know these things? Most assuredly, I say to you, 'We speak what we know and testify what we have seen, and you do not receive our witness. If I have told you earthly things and you do not believe, how will you believe if I tell you heavenly things?

No one has ascended to heaven but He who came down from heaven, *that is,* the Son of Man who is in heaven. And as Moses lifted up the serpent in the wilderness, even so must the Son of Man be lifted up, that whoever believes in Him should not perish but have eternal life. For God so loved the world that He gave His only begotten Son, that whoever believes in Him should not perish but have everlasting life. For God did not send His Son into the world to condemn the world, but that the world through Him might be saved. (NKJV)

Jon *hmphed*, shook his head, and shuffled to the door to prepare for the show. I've always felt a deep love for him. I have that video somewhere in my garage.

❦

Stuck on the set of *Andy's Rainbow* for ten hours at my doctor's desk, playing the head of the mental institution in Indiana, I had a lot of time to ruminate and doodle. There was a book about forgiveness right there on the desk. We were using a pastor's office. I read it while I waited for the lighting to be adjusted. The author was unable to forgive the man who murdered his grandmother. God asked him, "Are you *willing* to forgive?" The man answered, "Well, you commanded me to."

Then Peter came to Jesus and asked, "Lord, how many times shall I forgive my brother or sister who sins against me? Up to seven times?" Jesus answered, "I tell you, not seven times, but seventy-seven times" (Matthew 18:22).

"But if you do not forgive, neither will your Father who is in heaven forgive your transgressions."

Mark 11:26 NASB

Sometimes it's impossible to forgive others. I guess our flesh can't do it, but if we are filled with the Holy Spirit, maybe we can. We should ask God to help us forgive. It's not a trait that comes naturally to the flesh.

The author of the forgiveness book reluctantly tells the Lord he is *willing* to forgive but does not know how. First, the Lord asks him to pray for the murderer not to go to hell. The author reluctantly starts doing that. He can do that. Eternity is a long time. Then, the author realizes that in praying for the murderer not to spend eternity in hell, he is praying for the murderer to be in heaven, which means being born again, forgiven, and one of the family of God, his brother in Christ. Eventually, the feelings of hate turn into concern for the murderer's soul and his brotherhood.

Hmm. Well, that's one way to approach forgiveness, I guess. But, I don't think Husband is going to hell. He's just making me feel unloved.

One place we were filming was the apartment of a woman named Patsy. I was looking around, killing time. No crosses or Bible verse plaques. Then, I saw a framed photo of a man with wild curly black hair. I asked Patsy who it was.

Meher Baba—self-realization guru from India.

Uh oh.

Supposedly, he claims to be Jesus and God and every prophet. He keeps coming back as different amazing people, supposedly. He took a twenty-year vow of silence.

Well, I've got my work cut out for me. She actually believes a guy is God just because he says he is. He wasn't the theme of a book written over 2,000 years by at least forty-four different authors, some who never met yet have the same message, many who died for their eyewitness account of Him. Meher Baba wasn't miraculously born of a virgin. He didn't rise from the dead as reported by even nonbelievers like Josephus or do miracles or alter time—switching it from BC to AD. He didn't fulfill any prophecies written about him in the Torah thousands of years before his birth. He didn't live a perfect life. He just said, "I'm god."

And, she believes him?

Jesus warned us that false Christs and prophets would come and attempt to deceive even God's elect (Matthew 24; 2 Peter 3; Jude 17–18).

How can one recognize a false teacher or false prophet? The best way to guard ourselves against deception is to know the Truth. To spot a counterfeit, you must study the real thing. Jesus also said you will know a tree by its fruit (Matthew 12:33). They must admit Jesus is God. They must teach the gospel correctly—the death, burial, and resurrection of Jesus for forgiveness of sins. And does the teacher or prophet have the fruit of the Spirit? Characteristics that resemble Christ?

When I looked at Meher Baba's photo, my heart beat faster. I hate deceit. I hate deceit in politics, religion, marriage—everywhere.

I told Patsy I went to Bible college, and I would read Baba's literature skeptically and probably be reporting back to her proof as to why he is a liar.

She smiled back at me like the *Mona Lisa*.

I read the Meher Baba's book *Discourses* and concluded that it's trying to sound deep, but much of it is meaningless. He says things like, "He who knows everything displaces nothing." What? Baba's words are very insidious, tiny bits of biblical truth mixed with lots of lies. It's Oprah's religion and cancer-survivor Kris Carr's religion. It's New Age, and it's not just another false religion but the oldest, the first.

It was born in the garden of Eden. Satan as the serpent tempted Eve with the forbidden fruit by telling her if she ate it, she would be equal with God.

Baba teaches, "Whether man knows it or not, there is for him only one aim in life, and eventually he realizes this when he consciously experiences his own eternal and infinite state of 'I Am God.'"

Now this is mind candy. What a fun concept. If you are God, you make the rules. And, Jesus didn't have to die for your sins. There is no such thing as sin.

Patsy told me she reads the Bible too. She said you can believe both God's Word and Meher Baba. That is not true. They are opposite on many doctrines. Baba's ideas are from Satan, the enemy of God.

First of all, it's hard to put a label on Baba's belief system. He mentions yoga, a higher consciousness, self-realization, and then universalism when he says God is in the center of a circle and each religion is a spoke leading to the center, and all the spokes (religions) are the same and all of them lead to salvation and God.

Jesus says, "I am the way, the truth and the life; no one comes to the Father but by me" (John 14:6 NKJV).

Baba says, "The really happy are those who are always contented with their lot."

God through Solomon, the writer of Proverbs, says, "Godliness with contentment is great gain."

Baba says, "Try to be cheerful even in trying periods."

Jesus says through James, "Count it all joy when you fall into various trials" (James 1:2 NKJV).

Baba says, "True humility is strength, not weakness. It disarms antagonism and ultimately conquers it." Jesus says, "Anyone who wants to be first must be the very last, and the servant of all" (Mark 9:35).

And here are several more verses about humility:

- Luke 9:48: "For it is the one who is least among you all who is the greatest."
- James 4:10: "Humble yourselves before the Lord, and he will lift you up."
- 1 Peter 5:6: "Humble yourselves, therefore, under God's mighty hand, that he may lift you up in due time."
- Proverbs 11:2: "With humility comes wisdom."

Baba says, "For I tell you with divine authority, that God is Existence, eternal and infinite. He is Everything." [2]

That's a lie. God created everything, but He is not everything. God is not Satan. God is not my truck (Genesis 1 and John 1).

Romans 1 says that because of their sin and rebellion, God gave the people over to a lie and they worshipped the creation rather than the Creator.

Baba teaches reincarnation.

Jesus says, "And as it is appointed unto man once to die, but after this the judgment" (Hebrews 9:27 KJV). In other words, you don't die over and over, working your way up the ladder.

Many false prophets have tried to detract from or add to Scripture, including Mormon founder Joseph Smith, Islam founder Mohammed, Jehovah Witness founder Russell.[3] Only the Bible's message teaches that no amount of good works can make a person good enough to spend eternity with a holy God in a perfect place. Only the spotless Lamb, Christ, and His death on the cross can pay for our sin. Hallelujah!

I pray Patsy learns the Word well enough to know the difference between the true Savior and the fake Baba.

I'm still in awe of the kind-hearted families I'm working with, shooting this movie in the cornstalks of Indiana. It feels like time is fifty years behind here. People are polite, they wave, they go to church. I've always wanted to meet an Amish person, and yesterday was my big chance. I was licking a forbidden, potentially cancer-causing See's Lollypop in my hunting lodge room and saw a wheelchair guy and two young men in Amish attire walk briskly by my window.[4]

We had a nice conversation, and although I know it's rude, I asked for a photo with the Amish brothers. My paralyzed friend in the wheelchair (accidental gunshot wound from hunting buddies) volunteered to take the picture with his cell. A week later when I asked him to send it to my cell, he said he couldn't send it to me because he erased it out of respect for his Amish friends. They believe it's vain to take a photo of one's self. I had put them on the spot.

I wanted an excuse to visit a real Amish home. The two Amish brothers I met, Johnny and Menno, gave me the chance. Their mom sells flowers from their home. I found their address in my GPS. Almost felt guilty for using the technology. Met Eli, their dad, and asked him if Amish believe in works for salvation.

Eli: No. There are a lot of misconceptions about Amish, like, we don't pay taxes. We do.

Me: Why the horses and buggy? What Bible verse tells you to do that?

Eli: We just got used to this lifestyle from the old country.

Eli told me the history of the Amish. There was a split in Switzerland between the Swiss and Alsatian Anabaptists in 1693. Those who followed Jakob Ammann became the Amish. Those who followed Menno Simons became the Mennonites. They are all different: some liberal, some conservative, some use cell phones, some no phones. He said cell phones are a big temptation.

Later, on a cold and rainy day, I ran into Brother Menno at a gas station. I was in my warm car waiting for my gas tank to fill; he was filling up a can of gas in the cold rain wearing just a blue homemade shirt and black homemade vest. He got back in his horse and buggy and started trotting home. I passed him as he slowly clopped along home.

He's twenty-five with three kids already. In Los Angeles his good looks would make him a surfer dude/actor/model, but he was raised this way. He's humble and looks at the ground a lot. He has a twinkle in his eye and a curiosity. He has a slight lisp, and I noticed his dad, Eli, has the same lisp and though forty-eight looked thirty. Must be that clean living and the organic fruits and veggies in his garden.

I gave Eli forty-three dollars for the flowers. Weird Al's song was correct. They are self-sufficient—pigs, chickens, cows, their own milk, and veggies. Candles. Sewing. Home cooking. Neat, clean home. Big porch, big barn, horses. Nature. God. And their biblical doctrine is sound. I'm relieved. They are the closest to God.

I told Eli how much I admired their devotion to God.

Eli replied, "All religions have hypocrites."

I called Husband to see what he was doing at home without me for ten days. He listed all the Christian activities clearly and mumbled over the barhopping adventures with the millionaire.

Me: Barhopping!

Husband: Just smoking a cigar with friends.

Me: Semantics!

It made me physically ill and bitter in mind and spirit. Anger, hate, pain, and sadness washed over me. Same as the last twenty-three years. The men-only bar thing. It's wrong. It's not Christian. Freedom. I'm in the way of his freedom!

And now, I'm old, bald, flat, and sick.

I looked out at the rain in Salem, Indiana. This world is sad. Women are cheated on every day. People are not loyal. They lie. I think I'm a fun, optimistic, loyal person.

I texted Lannie. I asked for the number of a Christian divorce lawyer. He said he'll look, but he never does send me a number. He's praying for my marriage to last.

I hate being sad.

Live with a man who hates me and disrespects me? People do it all the time. That's one choice. Is there a companion out there who'd smile when I walked in a room? Who'd share secrets with me? Who'd put me first, above all others, male and female? Who'd try not to hurt me? Who'd make me laugh? Who'd love to hang out with me?

Back in the good ol' days I thought I was one of the lucky ones, the ones who don't get cheated on or lied to and who don't catch diseases like cancer because of our strong will, luck, optimism, and devotion to God.

> "Your Father in heaven … causes his sun to rise on the evil and the good, and sends rain on the righteous and the unrighteous."
> MATTHEW 5:45

I had a crying scene in a cemetery one day. I usually *cannot* cry on cue.

I texted my mom, *I had a crying scene today, and I did it!*

Mom texted back, *What did you think of to bring on the tears?*

Me: *Husband. And, Scarlet's two friends with young children who just got cancer. And my friend Danita who is in chemo now. And, what is the meaning of life. And, God.*

AOL news reports: "The team at Harvard Medical School calculated that twenty to forty percent of cancer cases, and half of cancer deaths, could be prevented if people quit smoking, avoided heavy drinking, kept a healthy weight, and got just a half hour a day of moderate exercise."[5]

My dad told me that fifty years ago.

Back from the movie, nursing my wounds from Husband's abandonment of me to play with his cigar buddies, I called a divorce lawyer. Then, my friend Leanne gave me a book entitled *The Love Dare* by Alex and Stephen Kendrick. It's a forty-day challenge about loving your spouse like Christ loves us—unconditionally. Loving someone who is mean to you.

I figured I would postpone divorce until I'd tried every last thing to save my marriage. On about day seven of the love dare, I asked Husband if I was being a good wife lately.

He thought about it and said yes.

I mumbled, "Well, it's killing me."

He looked amused.

One day I wondered, *Where's Husband? Didn't talk to him today once or see him.*

I think about him all the time. I must love him.

I just wish he loved me. I must be the loneliest girl in the world.

I'm pretty sure he only stays with me because he does not want to split his pension in half.

I wonder if we got divorced if I could fall in love with someone else. I'm so used to Husband's ways, and his body, his cough, his rumbly voice, his sour deadpan face, his tidiness, his paper towel placed next to the sink to hold his drink so that condensation drops don't touch the formica countertop that is made to get wet and not leave rings, his orderly rows in the refrigerator, his habit of sweeping the kitchen every night, his repulsion to playing the piano, even though he's really good at it, his repulsion to speak in public, his muscles, his smell …

Joke from my act:

My husband the cop is anal retentive, which is a good quality for a cop. He can always find the key to the hand cuffs. But, it drives me crazy. He even has a list in his wallet of things to do that he checks every day. And, on the list it even says, "Make list!" He has categories underlined like Personal, Car, Groceries …

I asked him, "Does Personal mean like brushing your teeth and going to the bathroom?" He didn't answer me. So, once I snuck in his wallet, and I wrote a new category, "Wife," and I underlined it. Under it I wrote, "Kiss her."

He found the note and said, "You're a nymphomaniac!"

I said, "I've never stolen anything in my life!"

Then, I got real brave and snuck in his wallet again, and under "Wife" I wrote, "Meaningful eye contact!"

I dream of a husband who would spend time with me, look me in the eyes without me asking, hug me without me begging, make love to me without me starting it, surprise me, travel with me, share hobbies, enjoy my perkiness, sleep next to me at night and have pillow talk. Wake up with me in the morning. A man who would love the outdoors and living in a log cabin.

One night, I pulled into my driveway at 11:00 p.m. after singing at Kimbro's, and Husband was there looking all handsome and muscular with his shirt tucked in and shoes on, smoking a cigar and reading the paper on the front porch. He gave me a nod.

If that is all the love I can get from him, it's something, I guess.

I was on the cell talking to redheaded Torry. As I negotiated my cell phone, my bra with the fake boobs in it (which I removed before exiting the car), my pearl necklace, shiny high heels, and my heavy purse, my Martin ukulele smashed into the pavement.

He came over and looked me in the eye. "Can I carry something?"

Well, this is new. It's a start. Meaningful eye contact. I found this note scribbled in my devotional from 2007:

Every time you push me away when I try to kiss you,
Every time you humiliate/punish me in public,
Every time your words slice the air and my heart,
You cut away another chunk of my bleeding soul,
And make the day closer when I can no longer forgive 70 x 7.[6]

Another night, Husband sweetly and romantically asked me to make love with him. He also bought me a dozen roses and a cute card for Mother's Day. I guess he figured it was an even exchange for choosing his buddies over me for ten days.

My jaw dropped. When I recovered from the shock, I started screaming expletives at him like an insane person.

I could not believe it. Husband has no clue. He actually doesn't know how much and how often he is hurting me.

When my heart quit racing, I calmly invited him into the Library/Jungle Room for a talk. He ate pasta while I told him that our marriage was horrible.

"For twenty-three years," he added.

I agreed. "We either have to get divorced or change something. This is not working."

Husband then proceeded to repeat my flaws, again, in full hate voice.

I sighed. "Every talk turns into this." Pause. "Let's get a divorce. Nothing is changing."

He then listed all of his great assets and why he is a wonderful person: "I pay all the bills. I clean the bathrooms …"

Clean the bathrooms? Clean the bathrooms!

That is not on my list of requirements for a husband. I don't want him to clean the bathrooms! I want him to love me.

He doesn't get it.

We live in alternate universes.

As the lonely night progressed, I found him beginning his cigar-smoking-reading-until-5:00-a.m.-on-the-porch ritual and calmly told him, "You were mean to me up there. Do you want to read the Bible?"

I started our nightly prayer and Bible reading ritual as a means to bring us closer to Christ and so to each other. It's my favorite time of day.

He came upstairs for the Bible ritual.

While he was reading the book of Joshua, I whispered, "I don't think we should get divorced."

He whispered back, "I don't either."

"Please don't bring up the past anymore. I'm highly educated on it. I already know it well. Unless it's something happy."

"Okay."

And, the bitter, painful, regret-filled, revenge-seeking twenty-three-year marriage full of resentment and tears continues to plod along like a weary horse whose owner has overworked and underfed him. Bruised, sad, and hopeless.

God can fix anything. I'll keep talking and walking with God. Maybe Husband will join us.

"Do you not know that your bodies are temples of the Holy Spirit, who is in you, whom you have received from God? You are not your own; you were bought at a price. Therefore honor God with your bodies" (1 Corinthians 6:19–20).

TIP: Try the Love Dare for 40 days before you give up on your marriage. Loving someone who is mean to you. Jesus loved us when we didn't love Him.

Lavender Hair

Gray hair is a crown of glory;
it is gained by living a godly life.

PROVERBS 16:31 NLT

*L*iving with the knowledge that you had cancer and that it may return is like living with lavender hair—everything is the same yet different.

You walk around, do the same chores and hobbies, but people look at you differently. Your friends and family and doctors have a little glint in their eye. They're thinking:

You could die soon; this may be the last Christmas together, your second to last birthday. Your medical chart has a box checked where it used to say none with a squiggly line from top to bottom. You are vulnerable. You are human. You are not indestructible. You have an expiration date.

You look in the mirror in the bathroom and you look the same. But, there are scars across your chest and no breasts or nipples. You are deformed. Nothing a nice baggy shirt couldn't hide, or a prosthesis. A *prosthesis!* When did that word enter my vocabulary?

You can still wear sexy outfits, but you know and your husband knows, and maybe everybody knows, that under the alluring dress is a mangled car accident of a chest. Hey! Since when do Christians wear sexy, alluring outfits? The Bible firmly teaches women to be modest. So, there's one good thing breast cancer did to me: made me modest— and humble.

Cancer makes you humble.

Little baby chick fuzz started sprouting out of my head. After being bald for six months, I was thrilled to have hair. Any hair. A centimeter grew in, and it was gray! I was grateful. But, it was gray!

Whaaa—?

I have died my hair blonde since I was fourteen, so I didn't really know what color my hair was. The roots were always brown. The gray must be the chemo poison. As it grew in, I tried to embrace my new look as an older, mature, wise woman. My hair looked like my husband's. They always say that couples who stay together a long time start to look like each other.

At my birthday party, my friend Judy remarked, "Your hair isn't gray! It's lavender!" She is always brimming over with love and trying to uplift everyone around her. Out of the corner of my eye I saw Husband nodding and agreeing with her: "It looks lavender! It looks lavender!" I thought of all the tiny moments of love in between the moments of hate when he had tried so hard to make me feel pretty during these last months of bandages, blood, and baldness. It inspired this song:

"Lavender Hair"

He sees me as zaftig not heavy
He hears me as wise and not dull
He thinks that I'm super terrific
When others think nothing at all
He sees me as funny not silly
And graceful as Fred Astaire
And he doesn't notice the gray, he says I have lavender hair.

He cleans up my mess in the kitchen
He irons his clothes and mine too
He's shy but he'll go on the dance floor
If that's what I want him to do

His kisses are soft and yet manly
He mentions me in his prayer
And he doesn't notice the gray, he says I have lavender hair.

All alone in the moonlight
Stars watch from above
One says, "They're starting to look alike."
The other says, "Could this be love?"

Sometimes he yells about money
And makes me feel small
But he is the only honey
I want to cuddle by the fire in the fall
I never said he was perfect
His romantic gestures are rare
But he doesn't notice the gray, he says I have lavender hair.[1]

Jokes from my act:

We're driving in the car together. Paul's side of the car is clean, because he's anal retentive, (laugh) has the new-car smell. My side of the car has magazines, tabloids, my laptop, my "act" I'm working on, sunflower seeds, a gardenia floating in water in the plastic drink holder, Diet Coke, water bottles, a Sugar Daddy I licked half of and laid the other half on the paper 'cause it's half the calories (laugh), bubble gum ...

I say, "Paul, can we adopt a baby?"

Paul: "Look at yourself and your careless, haphazard life-style. You can't even take care of yourself, put your safety belt on. (laugh) You're the kind of person who'll end up pushing a grocery cart under the overpass with your laptop and your 'act' in it and the other bums will say, 'There goes the neighborhood.'" (laugh)

I say, "I bring wonderful mayhem into your orderly rut of a life."

Paul: "The only realistic outcome to our marriage is that one of us, whichever slips into dementia first, will be victimized by the other from years of pent up rage and retaliation." (laugh)

Me: "Oh, that's good. Say that last sentence again."

The one thing that comforts me about my newly unsexy body is that my husband's behavior toward me hasn't changed. He was always this cold and unhappy with me even when I was young and thin, and had boobs and hair!

I'm a bit afraid of chemicals since cancer. I timidly dye my hair blonde again. Wincing.

Is outward beauty so important? What is beauty?

God consoles, He gives beauty for ashes. He will "comfort all who mourn … [and] bestow on them a crown of beauty instead of ashes, the oil of joy instead of mourning, and a garment of praise instead of a spirit of despair" (Isaiah 61:1–3).

TIP: "Make yourselves beautiful on the inside, in your hearts, with the enduring quality of a gentle, peaceful spirit. This type of beauty is very precious in God's eyes" (1 Peter 3:4 CEB). Maybe in your husband's eyes too.

Radiation: Barbie and Ken and a Big Machine

> "For I know the plans I have for you," declares the LORD, "plans
> to prosper you and not to harm you, plans to give you hope and
> a future. Then you will call on me and come and pray to me, and
> I will listen to you. You will seek me and find me when you seek
> me with all your heart."
>
> JEREMIAH 29:11–13

*F*inished mastectomy. Check. Finished Chemo. Check. Finished my movie. Check. Back to reality.

A doctor with a name like Adunkahasof Chakusatrospheklshek is assigned to me for my radiation, which is to begin ASAP in my four-part treatment of mastectomy/chemo/radiation/estrogen-blocking pill for life or five years, whichever comes first. Dr. Chak, as she is called, walks into the room. She slowly and carefully explains to me the benefits and risks of radiation. I already know them but appreciate her kind bedside manner and thorough explanation.

I should know what people are doing to my body. They are now going to burn holes in me. I was told that my skin may eventually become red, irritated, and/or burned on the outside. Inside, since my cancer was on the left side of my chest/breast, a machine will be burning holes through my chest, trying not to hit my lungs or heart. However, a piece of each will probably be scarred, and I must not smoke because I'll only have partial lung capacity. I must focus on healthy eating, because my heart has a 5 percent chance of heart disease in ten years.

This saddens me. I am allowing someone to damage my vital organs right when I need them most in my aging, weakening time.

When Dr. Chak leaves the room, I look up at God and say, "Kill me now. Kill me now." Why a slow death? A long, slow, ugly death. Marilyn Monroe did it best. She died before she got cancer or got old.

I go home and suck See's Lollypops and watch Mariel Hemingway's *Running from Crazy* about suicide, and then Maria Bamford's new Netflix series, *Lady Dynamite*, based on her mental illness. It was way too dirty. I'm still her fan though.

I didn't feel like having a good attitude that day. Especially since a great interview on Eric Metaxas' radio show gave me the confidence to call Ray Stevens and play my new song, "It's a Broken World, Baby," to his partner, Buddy. I expected an invitation to sing it on his new show but didn't get one ... yet.

I'm desperately craving human love and touching, so I try to cuddle Husband tonight even though I'm still hurting from the Indiana incident.

❦

The Internet says a suppressed immune system allows the growth of cancer. We all have cancer, but most people fight it off.

My friend Candy had MammoSite Radiation Therapy (RTS), and it only took five days, but I don't think that would work for me. It involves blowing up a balloon in the cancer site and putting radiation there, *blah, blah, blah*. I think since mine spread to the underarm lymph nodes, they told me I need the *Star Trek* gamma rays to slice through my heart and lung area for six weeks every day.

I don't know. This is not my area of expertise. Above my pay grade. "Not in my toolbox," the American Idol judges would say.

I am lying topless under this scary big radiation machine while soft music plays. The song is "Cheer Up, Sleepy Jean." *Hmmph.* Seventies music for middle-aged ex-homecoming queens. Burnt skin reminds me of my favorite Bible story—Shadrach, Meshach, and Abednego:

Shadrach, Meshach and Abednego replied to him, "King Nebuchadnezzar, we do not need to defend ourselves before you in this matter. If we are thrown into the blazing furnace, the God we serve is able to deliver us from it, and he will deliver us from Your Majesty's hand. But even if he does not, we want you to know, Your Majesty, that we will not serve your gods or worship the image of gold you have set up."

Then Nebuchadnezzar was furious with Shadrach, Meshach and Abednego, and his attitude toward them changed. He ordered the furnace heated seven times hotter than usual and commanded some of the strongest soldiers in his army to tie up Shadrach, Meshach and Abednego and throw them into the blazing furnace. So these men, wearing their robes, trousers, turbans and other clothes, were bound and thrown into the blazing furnace. The king's command was so urgent and the furnace so hot that the flames of the fire killed the soldiers who took up Shadrach, Meshach and Abednego, and these three men, firmly tied, fell into the blazing furnace.

Then King Nebuchadnezzar leaped to his feet in amazement and asked his advisers, "Weren't there three men that we tied up and threw into the fire?"

They replied, "Certainly, Your Majesty."

He said, "Look! I see four men walking around in the fire, unbound and unharmed, and the fourth looks like a son of the gods."

Nebuchadnezzar then approached the opening of the blazing furnace and shouted, "Shadrach, Meshach and Abednego, servants of the Most High God, come out! Come here!"

So, Shadrach, Meshach and Abednego came out of the fire, and the satraps, prefects, governors and royal advisers crowded around them. They saw that the fire had not harmed their bodies, nor was a hair of their heads singed; their robes were not scorched, and there was no smell of fire on them.

Then Nebuchadnezzar said, "Praise be to the God of Shadrach, Meshach and Abednego, who has sent his angel and rescued his servants! They trusted in him and defied the king's command and were willing to give up their lives rather than serve or worship any god except their own God. Therefore, I decree that the people of any nation or language who say anything against the God of Shadrach, Meshach and Abednego be cut into pieces and their houses be turned into piles of rubble, for no other god can save in this way."

Then the king promoted Shadrach, Meshach and Abednego in the province of Babylon. (Daniel 3:16–30)

Radiation is an interesting experience. I am greeted by friendly technicians, male and female, every day. They see me topless for fifteen minutes, then I leave. I've only been topless before for two people in my life—my two husbands. I feel like a stripper now. Over 150 people in the Vanderbilt system have seen me topless by now.

I must lie perfectly still on a metal table while a big machine first X-rays me to make sure I'm in the perfect position and then zaps me in pinpointed strategic areas. This is very difficult. The staying still part. First, I'm sure I'm going to sneeze, then I have an itch, then I need to take a deep breath, but I can't. If I do, the high-speed electronic zapper might zap my heart instead of the invisible cancer cell in my left chest wall.

I finally start to relax even though I'm topless and in a weird position with my head tilted to the right, away from the rays and my left arm over my head, pillow under my knees, feet tied, grabbing a handle, leaving my breast bone protruding. It's dark and cool. I don't hear the usual pops, zings, and burrs, so I speak out.

The technicians come out of their safe zone and into the radiation chamber to tell me they have to redo my X-rays, because I moved a tiny bit when I talked.

"Isn't it bad to have another X-ray?"

"It's a minimal amount of danger compared to the treatment."

Oh.

They leave the room, because the zapping was so dangerous.

How comforting. I like the noises of *zings* and *zaps* from deep within the silver steel *Starship Enterprise* that wraps around me. I feel like it is killing the cancer. Something positive is happening. Something is fighting for me. It might be my imagination, but it feels like I'm getting a sunburn inside my left chest. A warm, radiant healing touch.

I think this is mostly due to the sweet faces and spirits of my technicians: Jackie, Josh, and Jill. They make me feel safe. If I had a technician that was sloppy or rude, I would not feel safe. I wonder if they teach them that or if that's just the kind of people who go into the medical field—kind people who want to help others.

Radiation doesn't hurt. I have my first of thirty-three that day. The zap only took a few minutes. I can't get a straight answer. Is it nuclear? Gamma rays? Supersonic waves burning the cancer out of me?

The tall, handsome male nurse, Josh, says, "Not burning."

"Not burning."

"It kills the cancer cells," he says.

"And healthy cells too."

"Yes. No. It kills the cancer cells."

"When does my skin possibly get burned?"

"Two weeks from now."

"Won't I get scar tissue under my skin?"

"It will change the tissue a little bit. The doctor will tell you about it."

"Some people say it makes you tired."

"No. Most people keep going to work."

I don't know what they are talking about, my technicians Jill and Josh, but they look like Barbie and Ken. This whole cancer thing is surreal. I have no pain. Never felt better. They take my blood pressure and say it is that of a teenager.

This is strangely enjoyable. People are *caring* for me. Their faces look a bit worried about me.

I rack my brain. How can I make my death artistic or funny or meaningful? I know I'm just a statistic, but I can try to make my journey interesting. I want to leave these people with an anecdote they can tell people at a party when asked about the celebrities or fading celebrities they've worked on.

I feel now like the world is full of healthy, carefree people with hair, and then there's the rest of us—the bald, dying few who were singled out by God for punishment, or because He didn't like us, or was mad at us.

I saw a pretty woman leaving the building when I entered. We exchanged a look with each other and a sad, knowing smile. There is a pamphlet in the empty, clean, plush lobby with a list of cancer support groups. The last thing I want to look at or talk to is another cancer victim. I love my friends who treat me the same, as if nothing is different.

Lou Ann, the lady I babysat for when I was twelve, died of breast cancer as did my gymnastic teammate, my *SNL* castmate, and my wardrobe designer Rita at the *Lil Romeo* TV show. Sarah Cannon, aka Minnie Pearl, had breast cancer but lived to eighty-three and died of a stroke.

I think I'm getting fatter. The doctor told me chemo makes most women gain weight, as does the estrogen-blocking pill letrozole, which I'm required to take for five years. I'm told letrozole may cause hot flashes and it will weaken my bones, so I must take calcium with it.

I feel fat lying here naked in front of these two strangers. So, I pretend I'm a man. Men are always proud of their bodies no matter how fat or hairy they are.

I told Husband he didn't have to go with me to each radiation appointment, so in the lobby I ask him, "Why are you here?"

He could have said, *Because I love you.* Instead, he said, "Because *you're* here."

I guess it could mean the same thing.

I said, "I was in Indiana, and you weren't there."

Silence.

This whole cancer thing seems like a big, icky practical joke, and I'm getting tired of it and want it to end.

At my next doctor's visit, my newest oncologist, who looked like he had a hangover, almost gleefully told me to expect my node-less arm to contract lymphedema.

"Just kill me now," I said.

No one laughed.

He looked at me like I was a dying middle-aged woman, not an *SNL* alumna who just attended the forty-year *SNL* reunion in a cute black dress and took a selfie with Taylor Swift.

I took a happy pill at night for the second time—Ativan. I have lots of oxycodone and other medications under my bed, left over from my double mastectomy surgery. I haven't wanted or needed any of them. I've been trusting God and looking at the silver lining. But that same day, when I found out Husband had to go smoke cigars with the Fornicators *again*, my spirit sagged. I'm tired of trying to be grateful and fearless.

I can tell people feel uncomfortable when I'm in the room. Husband said my cancer is the elephant in the room.

"Why?" I said. "They're all going to die soon too."

Good Hamlet, cast thy nighted color off,
And let thine eye look like a friend on Denmark.
Do not forever with thy vailèd lids
Seek for thy noble father in the dust.
Thou know'st 'tis common. All that lives must die,
Passing through nature to eternity.[1]

The radiation did not hurt for the first fifteen times or so, but the skin got pinker and redder, and the last two weeks it was raw and tearing. The two Tylenol every four hours for two weeks kept the pain at bay and then one day, it was healed. There is a great balm called Aquaphor that really soothes burnt skin. I lathered it on day and night.

At my last radiation, I took photos with my beautiful radiation technicians who were so kind to me. At my request they had started playing The Mamas and the Papas and at the right volume, during my fifteen minutes of zapping. Sweet Nurse Vicki was giving my burned raw, red, and purple blistered chest one last look, when she presented me with a Certificate of Completion of Radiation, and we both knew it was silly.

But it was the first time I cried. It was an acknowledgment that this nine-month ordeal had been completed. I had retained a good attitude and done my best to obey the difficult instructions and endure the pain, all the while juicing carrots, spinach, and grapefruit, refraining from alcohol and cigarettes (of course) and limiting sugar. I let out a long sigh, the breath I'd been holding in.

Medical science had done its best to kill my cancer and prevent its recurrence. Now, it was up to God. God and me.

Anyway, Vicki the nurse hugged me and said, "You should be proud. You've been through a lot. Some people even have friends and family with balloons in the lobby to celebrate their last treatment."

I looked sadly at the ground. I knew my family wasn't in the lobby. My husband had been acting like he despised me, most recently telling me we could not go to the Smoky Mountains to celebrate the end of my treatment and my birthday, because it would cost money. I had offered to pay with my pension, and had made the reservation, but I cancelled when I realized how horrible it would be to be trapped in a gorgeous log cabin, overlooking breathtaking mountain views, with a man who did not want to be there.

I took my Certificate of Radiation Completion and opened the door to the lobby. There was my radiant thirty-year-old daughter, Scarlet, with a grin from ear to ear (it was her idea to surprise me), along with my five-year-old granddaughter, Ever Grace, who was holding helium balloons, and one-year-old Brooklyn Hope, who was reaching toward me desperately like I was the greatest person in the world. My mom and husband were standing there smiling sweetly. I was so surprised. I felt loved.

Maybe things will be going upwards from here.

I was asked to give my cancer testimony at church for a women's conference. I'm humbled and honored to get to share Jesus with a big group.

I visited Pretty in Pink, a mastectomy boutique, and the kind-hearted workers there suited me up in some really lifelike fake breasts you insert into a special bra with little slits that hold them in place. But, my skin was too tender to place any bra on, yet.

The whole invasion of privacy is almost unbearable except for the fact that it humbles me into knowing that we are all alike, vulnerable, scared, insecure, and never pretty enough. The kindness of these women in the prosthesis industry inspires me. I want to be like them. Their empathy wraps me in love and makes me feel okay about this whole thing. Many of them are breast cancer survivors, and they encourage me with their stories and gentle, knowing smiles.

In July 2016, I was on the *Alan Colmes Show* on the radio. He's very liberal, you know. There is a sweetness about him, though, when he's not talking politics. I thought the interview was about the presidential election—that's what his producer told me—so I was pleasantly surprised when Alan plugged my new song and YouTube music video, "It's a Broken World, Baby." Who knew that one could meet cancer and not only survive but thrive?

I had an urge from the Holy Spirit to share the gospel with Alan Colmes on the air, so I did. I had no idea that he was in treatment for lymphoma at the time until news of his death came February 23, 2017.

"It's a Broken World, Baby"

Tattoo of a broken ukulele
Light blue turquoise lies
He might leave me in the middle of my chemo
I would not be so surprised

Yeah, I got cancer and so does my dog
My car won't start and my sink has a clog
My checks are bouncing but my trampoline's torn
I am not surprised because I've been warned

It's a broken world, baby
I know you agree
The Second Law of Thermodynamics says
The world is in a state of entropy
That's a fancy word for broken you see

Lannie's back is causing him pain
Bob's OCD is driving Donna insane
Dilbert's dad, he needs a diagnosis
I quit kissing Daisy 'cause she has some halitosis

My heart is broken
Then I stubbed my big toe
I just got fired and
My food's GMO
I accidentally stepped onto my ukulele
Rushing to say hi to my new neighbor the Israeli
(well, you try to rhyme with ukulele)

It's a broken world, baby
Since Eve and Adam gave in

But there's a new world coming
That's why my song has a grin

Jesus is coming soon
Morning or night or noon
I'm gonna meet Him in the sky
In the twinkling of an eye[2]

I'm so sick of this medical stuff, I distract myself all day by writing new jokes for my next performance at Zanies Comedy Club. I want to attack the topic of cancer and death.

I just saw *Our Town* for my first time. There was a scene where a dead guy in the cemetery says, "We weren't just living. We were watching ourselves live."

Later someone says: "Yes, now you know. Now you know! That's what it was to be alive. To move about in a cloud of ignorance; to go up and down trampling on the feelings of those ... of those about you. To spend and waste time as though you had a million years. To be always at the mercy of one self-centered passion, or another. Now you know—that's the happy existence you wanted to go back to. Ignorance and blindness."

Musing on the 200 plus weddings he's performed, the pastor in *Our Town* says, "Once in a thousand times, it's interesting."[3]

Dr. Rexer gave me another checkup. I was happily surprised that they did not consider me metastasized. He said they count the lymph nodes and breast as the same thing and that it doesn't appear the cancer has spread to any other organs. Thank you, Jesus.

I'm trying to obey my own advice, and forget the past. So, I gave Husband a hug and a kiss. I'm sure this was a difficult journey for him too. I buried the long list of cruelties he dealt me.

He tried to wipe the hate from his face. His face was blank. It's carried hate on it for so long, he doesn't know what expression to paint on it now. His default face is disgust, indifference, or superiority. That day it looked confused. It will fall back into default face by night—angry.

I guess there is no marriage in heaven. Jesus said, "At the resurrection people will neither marry nor be given in marriage; they will be like the angels in heaven" (Matthew 22:30).

Maybe we spend too much time thinking about that stuff. *He loves me. He loves me not.* Two sinners cannot possibly have a perfect relationship here on broken earth. The apostle Paul encouraged believers to stay single and use their energy for spreading the gospel![4]

I saw my surgeon, Dr. Grau, for a checkup. She looked for lumps and didn't find any. Thank you, God.

I asked her how soon she could take my port out (surgically) and cut the little fat lumps off my sides.

She said, "Anytime for the port, but the plastic surgeon may want to leave the sides there for his breast reconstruction."

I don't think I want fake boobs. Been there, done that. Got the wet T-shirt.

This is my new normal. White halls. White coats. Lots of white plastic bottles with squirty antiseptic on the hallway walls. The medical staff squirt their hands before and after they touch me, every time. Like I have cooties.

Rejoice in the Lord always. Again I will say, rejoice! Let your gentleness be known to all men. The Lord is at hand. Be anxious for nothing, but in everything by prayer and supplication, with thanksgiving, let your requests be made known to God; and the peace of God, which surpasses all understanding, will guard your hearts and minds through Christ Jesus. Finally, brethren, whatever things are true, whatever things are noble, whatever things are just, whatever things are pure, whatever things are lovely, whatever things are of good report, if there is any virtue and if there is anything praiseworthy—meditate on these things. The things which you learned and received and heard and saw in me, these do, and the God of peace will be with you.

PHILIPPIANS 4:4–9 NKJV

I stumbled upon this on the Internet one day: "Fear, anger, and frustration can cause DNA to change shape, which may reduce quality expression. DNA shutdown can be reversed by feelings of love, joy, appreciation, and gratitude."[5]

Maybe my difficult marriage was a blessing. It distracted me from cancer.

Cancer was a black cloud hovering over me for a year. The cloud is gone.

Cancer humbles me. My sheer force of will cannot fix this, neither can my optimism, or my sunny disposition. I realize my weakness and total dependence on the mercy of God.

So I praise you, Lord. And thank you for this hope. You are my only hope. And you, Jesus, are all I need.

I think I'm okay with dying now.

My friend Danita died.

She was diagnosed with multiple myeloma two months ago and texted me just last week, *I'm thinking of you a lot. Are you going to die? Am I going to die?*

I always loved her directness.

I'd asked a friend if Danita knew the Lord. He said, "Oh yes, for a long time. She's in heaven. I can see her beautiful face lit up with joy at seeing Jesus' face." Maybe she's meeting my dad, who is coaching gymnastics in that golden gym with Maureen, his ex-gymnast, as his assistant. Maybe they're meeting my pastor's son Josiah who died at seventeen in a car accident.

I muse to myself that death isn't hard. You don't have to do anything to die. You don't have to be funny or pretty or skinny or make people laugh or applaud. Just do nothing, and it happens!

But it's not natural. God didn't invent it. "The thief comes only to steal and kill and destroy" (John 10:10). It's Satan's idea, that's why its creepy.

In a way, this is my greatest performance! Dying.

Everyone is watching. Will I do it gracefully? Will I be a coward and swallow a bottle of pills? Will my faith be strong and apparent? Will I be funny? Will I write a song about it? A one-woman show? Will it be fast or slow? Will I be selfish and pity myself? Will I be mad at God? Or will I be anxious to see Him? Will I accept God's time or fight it? Will I be grateful and full of peace?

I hope I will be excited about this ultimate adventure.

If God lets me live fifteen more years like King Hezekiah, will I use the time for God's glory? Will I live it for Him?

Husband and I walk down to CeCe's Frozen Yogurt with my friend Jenny.

I mention death, and how I am tired of thinking about it.

Beautiful Jenny suggests, "Why don't you focus on how you can be a blessing to others?"

It was God speaking through Jenny to me.

My face lit up. That is what I will focus on. *Others.* That has always been the key to happiness. "Love the Lord thy God with all thy heart, and with all thy soul, and with all thy mind. … And, love thy neighbor as thyself" (Matthew 22:37, 39 KJV).

There was a spring in my step as we walked to the car.

I looked at my husband as he quietly drove us home. *I think I'll start with him.* Then I said, "Aren't my friends the greatest people?

Husband said yes.

"I wish you had friends like mine, instead of Cigar Brian, who just knocked up a Hooters' waitress," I said with disgust.

And, we drove home in silence.

I shouldn't have said that.

Praise be to the God and Father of our Lord Jesus Christ, the Father of compassion and the God of all comfort, who comforts us in all our troubles, so that we can comfort those in any trouble with the comfort we ourselves receive from God. (2 Corinthians 1:3–4)

TIP: It's a broken world, baby! Since Eve and Adam gave in. But there's a new world coming, and that's why my song has a grin.

ATHEISTS

> Now there are some things we all know,
> but we don't take'm out and look at'm very often.
> We all know that something is eternal. And it ain't houses
> and it ain't names, and it ain't earth, and it ain't even the stars …
> everybody knows in their bones that something is eternal, and
> that something has to do with human beings. All the greatest
> people ever lived have been telling us that for five thousand years
> and yet you'd be surprised how people are always losing
> hold of it. There's something way down
> deep that's eternal about every human being.
>
> —THORNTON WILDER, OUR TOWN

*I*n a debate with atheist Christopher Hitchens, Dinesh D'Souza points out that it takes faith to believe and it takes faith to deny.

In his 2010 Toronto debate with Tony Blair, Hitchens said, "Once you assume a Creator and a plan, it makes us objects in a cruel experiment whereby we are created sick and commanded to be well … and over us to supervise this, is installed a celestial dictatorship, a kind of divine North Korea [audience laughed here] … greedy for uncritical praise from dawn till dusk, and swift to punish the original sins with which it so generously gifted us, in the very first place. However, let no one say there is no cure. Salvation is offered, redemption indeed is promised at the low price of the surrender of your critical faculties."

Though clever and smug, Hitchens' opening remarks contain glaring errors to a Bible student like me. First of all, humans were not created in sin. According to Genesis, we were created perfect but with a free will, and we chose to disobey the Creator who made us. We chose to disbelieve His warning. We chose sin. So the rest of Hitchens' argument is faulty. It is based on a false premise.[1]

I compare myself to Hitchens. We look like the same person when we are both chemo bald. We both like writing, speaking to an audience, thinking about God, and imbibing.

Hitch died of esophageal and lymph node cancer at age sixty-two. He drank and smoked. Also, his father drank and died from esophageal cancer.

Hitch described his cancer as "taking me from the country of the well across the stark frontier that marks off the land of malady."[2]

In an interview, Charlie Rose brought up the smoking and drinking. And, Hitch said he was lucky to have lived a life of travel, books, language, and bohemia, but "if I'd have known I'd live this long, I would have taken better care of myself."

Rose: If you had known that there was a possibility of getting cancer, you would have never smoked a cigarette, you would have never consumed the amount of liquor you consumed.

Hitch: No, I think all the time I felt that life is a wager, and that I probably was getting more out of leading a bohemian existence as a writer than I would have if I didn't. So, and writing is what's important to me, and anything that helps me do that or enhances and prolongs and deepens and sometimes intensifies argument and conversation is worth it to me, sure.

Rose: What is the worst part of living with cancer? It puts some sense of mortality in your focus?

Hitch: No, because I think the focus on mortality is a useful thing to have.

Hitch: You want to know what the worst thing about it [cancer] is? I think the feeling that I'm boring.

Rose: Which your mother said was the worst sin.

Hitch: Yes, the unforgivable one.

Hitch: What else is bad about it? Makes you feel sick, time passes very slow, everything takes a long time, you never get the feeling you've done a full day's work, if you've done anything at all you're pleased, so your standards fall.

Rose: Has any of this caused you to have any change of your ideas or opinions about religion?

Hitch: No, why could it possibly do that?

Rose: Because of the old maxim that there are no atheists in foxholes.

Hitch: People who say, "Well, if you'd only give up the principles you've been attached to for a lifetime, you might impress God that way." The likelihood that intercessionary prayer or things of this kind are going to make a difference to you, whether you're healthy or ill seems to me to be nill.

Rose asked Hitch if he minds Christians praying for his conversion or salvation.

Hitch: Anyone who's kind enough to express sympathy, I'm not going to sneer at them no, that would be cheap … But there is a long, unattractive history of religious people going around claiming that nonbelievers reconsidered everything at the last and were received into the bosom and so forth.

He said he had no anger about death, but it looks as if he left the party earlier than he would have liked. I think Hitchens is verbose but not wise. "The fool has said in his heart there is no God" (Psalm 14:1).[3]

The god of this world (Satan) hath blinded the minds of them which believe not, lest the light of the glorious gospel of Christ who is the image of God, should shine unto them.

2 CORINTHIANS 4:4 KJV

The amazing and wonderful Steve Martin, who I got to work with on *SNL*, once said, "It's so hard to believe in anything anymore.

I mean, it's like, religion, you really can't take it seriously, because it seems so mythological, it seems so arbitrary … but, on the other hand, science is just pure empiricism, and by virtue of its method, it excludes metaphysics. I guess I wouldn't believe in anything anymore if it weren't for my lucky astrology mood watch."[4] In a piece for *The New Yorker* in 1998, entitled "Does God Exist?" Steve wrote, "Once you allow impossible ideas to coexist in your brain, you are on your way to being a very fine beast of burden. … Whatever answer you choose at any given moment is the correct one."[5]

Sounds agnostic. *Agnostic*: without knowledge.

I don't think Steve has read the entire Bible. There is something powerful that happens when one actually reads and ponders that book. And, maybe Steve equates the heavenly Father with his earthly father who is reported to have been very stern, critical, and not emotionally open.[6] In his clever song "Atheists Don't Have No Songs," Steve expresses in a funny way the sad truth that atheists really don't have anything to sing about.[7]

I got saved at age six. Was I brainwashed at Carol City Baptist Church? I remember the building with its cool dark cement hallways. The folding chairs and cheap ceiling of white rectangles with holes poked in them. The red velvet chairs on the pulpit. The heavy wooden stand and carved table with the open Bible on it.

The three services our family attended each week were orderly, repetitive, and respectful. There was love and peace in the air along with God's Word. It felt like truth—ageless, comforting, a rock. I was told this was the absolute truth, and I believed it.

And I still do.

Christians were humble. They admitted their sins, asked forgiveness, and tried to live better. Everyone had a testimony of how they came to know Jesus. The testimonies were so different—some wildly exciting, some not. But they always ended the same—at the cross.

My earliest memories are hearing about the blood of the Lamb, the crucifixion, death, the afterlife. I found comfort in the fact that these people were confronting reality, not ignoring it, or numbing themselves, not lying about it, or dolling it up like a TV show comedy, not ignoring the facts—the inevitability of death, the constant struggle with sin, and the required redemption and hope.

It's been ten days since radiation ended, and my chest still burns and hurts. I'm taking two to three Advil every four hours. It's healing slowly. Occasionally there's a sharp pain in the place where the cancer was exhumed, and I fear it is still growing there.

I don't want to die now. There, I finally admitted it.

Dr. Adrian Rogers says, "Faith is a gift from God, but does that mean if God gives faith that we are going to automatically believe? No.

Just like faith is a gift from God, breathing is a gift. God gives me lungs and air, but I can smother if I want to."[8]

Whosoever will, let him take the water of life freely.

REVELATION 22:17 KJV

But we have this treasure in earthen vessels, that the excellence of the power may be of God and not of us. *We are* hard-pressed on every side, yet not crushed; *we are* perplexed, but not in despair; persecuted, but not forsaken; struck down, but not destroyed—always carrying about in the body the dying of the Lord Jesus, that the life of Jesus also may be manifested in our body.

2 CORINTHIANS 4:7–10 NKJV

I'm lying in the surgical unit of Vanderbilt University Medical Center in Nashville looking at my texts. They are taking my port out today. Hopefully, I won't need it ever again.

Husband is sitting nearby, and Rachel Ray is cooking on the TV overhead.

Procedures are my new normal. I'm not nervous. I tell Husband that if I die during surgery to give Aubrey the butter mints in my purse that I got for her during William's wedding. She loves butter mints. She'll know I was thinking of her.

Husband mumbles, "You're not going to die."

"Next year I'll have hair and boobs. Will you still be around? Are we getting divorced?"

Husband shakes his head. "Too much invested."

I look at my texts. Scarlet writes, *Ever woke up this morning and said, "I miss Bam Bam. Does she still have cancer?"* I smile.

Then, I see a video from the two of them. Scarlet is at the piano singing a sincere original song she wrote about adopting their new deaf baby girl from China. It's called "Joy Comes in the Morning." They named Wang Ya Zhu "Joy." (Side note: Joy, age four, who could not walk, began to walk alone two weeks after they adopted her. Also, with a device from Vanderbilt on her hairband, she can now hear! She also learned twenty sign language signs in the first week. Mostly, the sign for *food*. She was starving. Not anymore. God is so good!)

Blue cap, hospital gown, ugly hospital socks, clean floors, I'm lying on the rolling bed. I could get used to this. The drugs are good. I'll have a great nap.

Suddenly, I'm waking up. I have a slightly euphoric feeling. Anything else I could get cut off? I want another hit.

Job said, "Naked I came from my mother's womb, and naked I shall return there. The Lord gave and the Lord has taken away. Blessed be the name of the Lord" (Job 1:21 NASB).

TIP: Listen to God. He has the "words of eternal life" (John 6:68).

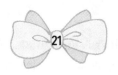

Zanies:
ALMOST One Year Later

Many are the plans in a person's heart,
but it is the LORD's purpose that prevails.

PROVERBS 19:21

This cancer experience gave me a fresh attitude, a new gratitude, a
rush of energy, and enthusiasm for life. I'm still here. My cancer
treatment is all done. And I know that God determines when and if
I will die. Maybe I'll be the generation who sees Him coming in the
sky and gets caught up in the clouds to be with Him. Maybe I can skip
death and just walk on up to heaven like Elijah and Enoch.

Cancer didn't make me find God. I'd found Him long ago. But,
cancer did rearrange my priorities a bit; cancer is not at the top, Jesus
is, staying healthy second, marriage next, and then seeking God's will,
one day at a time.

Trivial worries don't bother me anymore. I have hair! I'm so happy
to have hair again, nothing bothers me. The memory of being in my
bed in the fetal position, so weak with the Red Devil chemo that all I
could do was talk to God and listen to Debi Selby sing "River of My
Life" over and over and how that was enough and I was actually happy
like that, encourages me to tackle any mountain.

Little stuff doesn't matter. I just auditioned for a TV show and got
rejected. It used to worry me a lot. Now, *pfft*! I have hair! And, I feel
great. No cough! Life is wonderful.

I ask Brian, the owner of Zanies, for a date to do my stand-up act again even though my hair is gray and barely there. I want to mark this remarkable season of life with a celebration show. It's 2016, a year after my diagnosis. He books me.

I am curious how doing a show in my current state will feel psychologically. Will I be more relaxed? Now that my priorities are different? Bombing onstage is nothing compared to life and death.

I do the show. I am relaxed, I have a great time. I'm not coughing. I do my new cancer jokes! My friends fill the room and pour waves of love on me. And, standing ovations!

I wear a fluffy blonde wig with a big bow, and in the middle of the set, I dramatically take it off to reveal my gray crew cut to great applause. I joke, *"My husband says I look like an 'Androgynous drill sergeant'" (big laugh)*. I sing my new song, "Lavender Hair," and tear up a bit, and the audience does to.

A two-time Emmy winner producer happens to be in the audience that night, and she loves my set. I tell her my idea of a semi-reality TV show about an *SNL* alum who's living in Nashville and decides the last unchecked thing on her bucket list is to sing her original ukulele songs at the Grand Ole Opry. Her only obstacles: (1) her age, (2) cancer, and (3) her voice! Everyone loves a good comeback tale! I am now pitching this to the networks, and I'm "playing out" around town, doing what I love best: trying to make people laugh.

> Even though our outward man is perishing, yet the inward man is being renewed day by day. For our light affliction, which is but for a moment is working for us a far more exceeding and eternal weight of glory, while we do not look at the things which are seen but at the thing which are not seen.
>
> 2 CORINTHIANS 4:16 NKJV

My small group literally prayed me through the valley of the shadow of death. They laid hands on me and prayed hard when they heard I had cancer. Over the year, they watched me go bald and then watched my hair and energy come back. The love of Christ pouring through them was a rock for me. Praying for their needs reminded me that I am not the only one with hardships.

My Bible group leader, Lannie the lawyer, danced at a Bar Mitzvah with John Travolta—that is cool. We also have a doctor, a homemaker, a realtor, an ex-stripper, a pharmacist, a dog groomer, a retired helicopter police pilot/SWAT guy, an actress, and a Welsh sailor who travels the world looking for oil in the oceans on a ship with an all Muslim crew. I love my group.

Trying to keep my marriage together all these years has been a tougher fight than cancer. Emotional pain is worse than physical pain. And human love is elusive.

When I was a child and heard that all the commandments could be reduced to two: (1) love God with all your heart, soul, and mind and (2) "love your neighbor as yourself" (Matthew 22:36–40). I thought that was easy. It was only after years of life that I began to understand how impossible those two commandments are to keep. All the more reason we need a Savior.

I asked Husband one day, "Why am I happy about dying again? I forgot."

Without missing a beat, he replied, "You're reading that heaven book."

"Oh yeah."

"And there's a Starbucks there," he says deadpan.

You see, that's why I just have to love him, despite everything. He's so funny.

When Paul and I were telling my girlfriends how my breast cancer was diagnosed, I whispered, "I went in for a cough, had a numb spot, *blah, blah, blah*. I thought my breast implants were slipping or something. They were twenty-five years old."

Husband interjects, "You had breast implants?"

Everyone laughs for a full five minutes.

The good thing about having a death sentence (we all do, but cancer victims are more aware of it) is that you use that special pink rose china you were saving for the future for a special time, you wear that silk top in the back of your closet that is impossible to wash so you were saving it for a special occasion, you tell the nail technician named Willis about Jesus. It may be your last chance.

We are characters in the plot of His story, so lucky to be included, created by Him to be in His story. History.

God teaches me something new every time I open the Bible.

How did people hear from God before there was a Bible? The same way we hear God today. God speaks to us. He speaks in many different ways to those who want to hear Him: audibly, inaudibly, in person, in dreams, in visions, through other people, and through the Bible.

"The joy of the LORD is your strength."
NEHEMIAH 8:10

This cancer diagnosis is a lifelong thing. Currently it means I'll have to take the estrogen-blocking pill letrozole every day. I feel no major side effects so far—just a dry-ish mouth, a hint of a hot flash occasionally. I'll be visiting the breast clinic every three months, then every six months, then every year, then every three years for checkups.

Dr. Rexer asks if I'll volunteer for an experimental drug, but I decline. Half of the test patients get a placebo, the other half a pill that is supposed to kill cancer that sometimes sneaks around the letrozole (this is scientific research, testing, but the side effect is mouth sores and I can't bear to think of one more discomfort).

Dr. Rexer said that my five months of chemotherapy, thirty-three radiation treatments, and the double mastectomy rid my body of every cancer cell they could see: "If there is any cancer left, it is invisible."

I have a thought bubble hovering over me: "If it happened once, it can happen again."

If it returns, and I have to go through treatment again, and again, as some cancer patients do, I'll have more people to tell about Jesus. If I die of a heart attack next year as a side effect from the radiation on my left side, even better. I will be with Jesus. With God.

Cancer is not a death sentence. Birth is. Everyone is dying. Jesus died. He showed us how. If God can go through death, I can. Of course, He rose again from the grave, showing me that I can do that too. This hope is fantastic.

This is the joy Christians carry around with them.

Each one of us is unique as a snowflake, as a thumbprint. Each one of us has an original DNA. We each have our own adventure, our own unique story, known by God before we were born.

A musician in Nashville, Bob Farnsworth, told me that his son was intimidated to play the guitar after this old jazz great. They were in the studio making a commercial. The jazz great said, "Go ahead. Strum it. No one in the world plays that song exactly like you do."

I am "fearfully and wonderfully made" (Psalm 129:14 KJV) and God knows the plans He has for me, "plans to prosper" me (Jeremiah 29:11).

My life and death are unique, and so are yours.

I heard God talk to me once in Los Angeles, around 1995 when I was sitting alone on Venice Beach at 9:00 a.m. one morning when I'd missed my plane and was in a deep depression over the state of my life. After I poured my heart out to Him, face full of tears, I heard Him say, "You want to control your life."

"Yes, I do."

He said again, "You want to control your life."

I replied out loud, "Yes, and I'm doing a pretty good job. I got famous, have a great family, bought a house or two."

He said again, "You want to control your life."

Looking out at the immense Pacific Ocean, I replied, "I lost all my money in a divorce. I drink too much, have a terrible marriage, a dead career, am sad, frustrated all the time ..."

"Or, I could control your life," God said, "I who made the ocean you're looking at and can't see to the other side, I who made the strange creatures in it, I who started the hearts beating in the babies in your stomach, I who created the people walking behind you. Or, I could control your life."

I knew all the church clichés. But this seemed like a real conversation between me and God. Very real.

"Okay," I said. "Control me. How does that work? Like a puppet? I mean, I have to stand up and walk away right now, back into life."

"Go home and love your family, and I'll tell you what to do."

That was it. *Boom.*

It was a powerful moment. I ran to tell my brother James at his nearby architectural office about my encounter. He said he believed me, because I was glowing.

So now, years later after surviving this big, scary cancer monster, I'm listening for God to talk to me again. I think He's saying: "Walk with me. You have great adventures ahead of you, just around the corner. It will be exciting and safe."

Recently at Music City Baptist, I heard a song by Lari Goss for the first time, sung by the precious Pastor Ben Graham, called "I Bowed on My Knees and Cried Holy." In it, Goss dreams about the gates of heaven and the angels who meet him there. First, he sees mansions and other wonderful sights. But then, the person he wants to see is the One who gave His life for me—Jesus.[1] I want it sung at my funeral (by Ben Graham if he's available)! There is only one person who ever died for me or who ever claimed to die for me. That's big. I want to meet Him.

I saw the LORD, high and exalted, seated on a throne; and the train of his robe filled the temple. Above him were seraphim, each with six wings: With two wings they covered their faces, with two they covered their feet, and with two they were flying. And they were calling to one another: "Holy, holy, holy is the LORD Almighty; the whole earth is full of his glory." (Isaiah 6:1–3)

TIP: Walk with God. "His mercies are new every morning" (Lamentations 3:23).

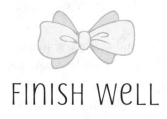

FINISH WELL

That is why, for Christ's sake, I delight in weaknesses,
in insults, in hardships, in persecutions, in difficulties.
For when I am weak, then I am strong.

2 CORINTHIANS 12:10

"*W*ell done, good and faithful servant" (Matthew 25:23). Every time I say that verse I cry. It's very powerful. I can't imagine Jesus would ever say that to me. I'm not a good enough servant. I've been too distracted and selfish. I've doubted His love and His word too many times. If He gave me a crown, I'd just lay it at His feet. What an honor that would be. His holiness is so beautiful to me.

I was in a college class at PBA (Palm Beach Atlantic University) in 2007 where I was finishing the BA degree I'd started thirty years before. You know, things got in the way. *SNL* ... raising babies. The teacher said, "What good is a life lived for God if you don't finish well? Finish well." The apostle Paul said, "I have finished the race, I have kept the faith, finally there is laid up for me the crown of righteousness" (2Timothy 4:7–8 NKJV).

I just got uninvited from a Christian talk show because they disagreed with my stand on some biblical issues and doctrine. I could cave, not lose career opportunities and friends. But 2 Timothy warned us against false teachers. I told them in a loving way why I thought they were doctrinally incorrect, and they never called back.

Recently, I was singing with my uke at a local cafe.

My husband says I sing like a bird—a screech owl.

Husband helped me write that joke.

That night in bed:

"Are you going to leave me?"

"No."

"Why?"

"We have too much history. Where would I ever find another you?"

"Aw. Are you going to cheat on me with a younger woman?"

"No. An older one."

"Ha-ha. No, really."

"No. I couldn't. You're everything I need and more. Way, way, way, way more. By about fifteen personalities."

"That's romantic."

"Because you're prettier than every other woman in the world, younger and older."

"Okay, okay, now you're just ..."

Maybe not today, maybe not tomorrow, but one day, God will heal all of us completely and forever.

Being confident of this very thing, that He who has begun a good work in you will complete it until the day of Jesus Christ.
PHILIPPIANS 1:6 NKJV

Job exclaimed, "Though he slay me, yet will I trust in him."
JOB 13:15 KJV

Forgetting those things which are behind, and reaching forth unto those things which are before, I press toward the mark for the prize of the high calling of God in Christ Jesus.
PHILIPPIANS 3:13–14 KJV

Nancy Missler wrote: "Faith comes in the form of a constant choice. A choice we can never stop making, no matter how hard the situation and no matter how long it lasts or who it involves. It's a choice to follow God and do what He asks, regardless of how we feel, what we think, or what we want."[1] Missler, age 77, just died from skin cancer that started as a bump in her nose.

It's interesting to me that Woody Allen is probably lying in bed in the dark tonight and like me thinking about death. I wish he knew God like I do.

I am healed. Cancer is a million miles away. Last year feels so long ago. I look down at my saddle shoes and smile. I'm writing a new song with my friend Jim ("But, I Do") for my youngest daughter's wedding. I'm bursting with joy.[2]

Will cancer come back? Will my husband leave me? Will my next marriage therapist explode? Will I live fifteen more years? What will I do with that time?

I'll walk with God. He is holding me with His right hand.

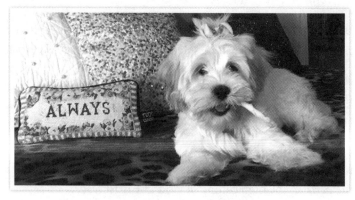

Our new puppy, Hezekiah.

Author's Note

As my great editors, Bill and Ocieanna, and myself untangled, organized, edited, and re-edited my messy year-of-cancer diary, I had to relive my cancer adventure. I don't like to think about it. But, it's encouraging to add another big answered prayer to my long list of victories in Jesus.

Daisy the Maltese died at age thirteen during the completion of this book. I think dogs go to heaven, so I look forward to seeing her again. Hezekiah, our new puppy, keeps me busy throwing her squeaky toy, thus effectively curtailing my See's Lollypop consumption.

Right now, I'm working on a Pureflix sitcom series and preparing for another Zanies performance. It's scheduled for October 8, 2017, exactly two years after my coughing Zanies date when I began the cancer journey. It will be a celebration of life and healing, a cancer research fund raiser in association with the Breast Cancer Research Foundation, and a book launch for this book, *Lavender Hair*, which I hope will comfort and remind others that they are not alone and God is still good.

ABOUT THe AUTHOr

Victoria Jackson is best known for her six seasons on *Saturday Night Live*, 1986–1992, and has also appeared in many films. Vicki was raised in a Bible-believing, piano-playing home with no TV. Her father was a Baptist deacon, ex-vaudevillian, and gymnastic coach, so she competed in gymnastics from age five to eighteen.

While at college on a gymnastics scholarship, Vicki discovered drama. An audition put her in contact with Johnny Crawford (*The Rifleman*) who promptly put her in his nightclub act and gave her a one-way ticket to Hollywood. Vicki supported herself by typing at the American Cancer Society, waitressing at The Kipling Retirement Home, and being a cigarette girl at the Variety Arts Center where Johnny Carson's talent scout saw her six minute stand-up comedy act and put her on *The Tonight Show Starring Johnny Carlson* where she appeared over twenty times.

In 1992 Vicki was reunited with her high school sweetheart, Paul Wessel, and left show business to raise a family in the suburbs of Miami. In 2007 she finished her B.A. in Film at Palm Beach Atlantic University.

Vicki still performs stand-up comedy and appears in an occasional film. She and her husband now reside in Nashville, Tennessee, to be near their daughters and grandchildren.

Connect with Victoria at VictoriaJackson.com,
Facebook.com/VictoriaJackson, Twitter.com/VictoriaJackson,
and Instagram.com/victoria_jackson_official.

NOTES

Devotional 5

1 Friedrich Nietzsche's anti-God philosophy permeated the sixties and helped switch American values from biblical morality to amoral relativism, secular humanism, a "do what feels good" ethic, the breakup of the family unit, and the "what's good is evil and evil is good" (Isaiah 5:20) chaos of today. Joni Mitchell named her cat Nietzsche.

2 Find the rest of my song on my website: victoriajackson.com.

Devotional 7

1 Victoria Jackson, "I Am Not a Bimbo." I sang this at the Update Desk on *SNL* in 1986 during the Steve Martin/Sting show. Find the rest of the song on my website: victoriajackson.com.

Devotional 8

1 In C. S. Lewis, *The Weight of Glory* (San Francisco: HarperCollins rev. ed., 2001), n.p.

Devotional 9

1 "Doxorubicin," *Wikipedia*, https://en.wikipedia.org/wiki/Doxorubicin.

2 "Cyclophosphamide," *Wikipedia*, https://en.wikipedia.org/wiki/Cyclophosphamide.

3 Find the rest of my song on my website: victoriajackson.com.

4 Excerpt from my chemo diary.

5 Excerpt from my chemo diary.

6 Excerpt from my chemo diary.

Devotional 10

1 Excerpt from my chemo diary.

2 James Andrew Miller and Tom Shales, *Live from New York: The Complete, Uncensored History of Saturday Night Live as Told by Its Stars, Writers, and Guests* (Little, Brown, 2014), n.p.

3 See, for example, *Burzynski, the Movie—Cancer Is Serious Business* (Eric Merola, 2009) and *The Health Show—Dr. Stanislaw Burzynski: Treating Brain Cancer with Antineoplastons*.

Devotional 11

1 Mary Steenburgen, *Parenthood*, directed by Ron Howard (Universal Studios, 1989), quoted in Mary Farrell and Vicki Sheff, "After Years on the

Mommy Track, Mary Steenburgen Knows the Full Route of Parenthood," *People*, August 28, 1989, http://people.com/archive/after-years-on-the -mommy-track-mary-steenburgen-knows-the-full-route-of-parenthood -vol-32-no-9/.

2 Victoria Jackson, "An Old Stamp," published in Florida Bible College newsletter (1976).

3 Excerpt from my chemo diary.

4 Psalm 23 (KJV).

5 Excerpt from my chemo diary.

6 Excerpt from my chemo diary.

7 Anne Graham Lotz, *Why? Trusting God When You Don't Understand* (Thomas Nelson, 2005), 25.

8 Ibid., 26.

Devotional 12

1 Excerpt from my chemo diary.

2 Excerpt from my chemo diary.

Devotional 13

1 Excerpt from my chemo diary.

2 John Piper, "Embrace the Life God Has Given You," Desiring God, http:// www.desiringgod.org/embrace-the-life-god-has-given-you.

3 Excerpt from my chemo diary.

4 Excerpt from my chemo diary.

5 "Exposure to Chemicals in Plastic," Breastcancer.org, http://www.breast cancer.org/risk/factors/plastic.

6 Excerpts from my chemo diary.

7 Find the rest of the song on my website: victoriajackson.com.

Devotional 14

1 Excerpt from my chemo diary.

2 Joyce Kilmer, "Trees," *Poetry*, https://www.poetryfoundation.org /poetrymagazine/poems/12744/trees.

3 Rudyard Kipling, "If—", *Poetry*, https://www.poetryfoundation.org /poems/46473/if---.

Devotional 15

1 Alanna Ketler, "Chlorine Is Toxic: What You Need to Know About Chlorine and Your Health," *Natural Blaze*, August 15, 2013, http://www. naturalblaze.com/2013/08/chlorine-is-toxic-what-you-need-to-know .html.

2 Alanna Ketler, "Chlorine in Water Could Be Linked to Human Cancers," *Collective Evolution*, August 15, 2013, http://www.collective-evolution. com/2013/08/15/chlorine-is-toxic-what-you-need-to-know-about -chlorine-your-health/.

3 Quoted in Ketler, "Chlorine Is Toxic."

4 Quoted in Ketler, "Chlorine in Water."

5 Excerpt from my chemo diary.

6 I wrote this song in 1983 and sang it on *The Tonight Show Starring Johnny Carson*. Find the rest of the song on my website: victoriajackson .com.

Devotional 16

1 "Turmeric," RxList, http://www.rxlist.com/turmeric-page2/supplements. htm.

2 Read William J. Boykin et al, *Shariah: The Threat to America* (Center for Security Policy, 2010).

Devotional 17

1 Excerpt from my movie diary.

2 The above quotes were taken from Maher Baba, *Discourses* (1967; San Francisco, CA: Sufism Reoriented, 1973).

3 Read *The Kingdom of the Cults* by Walter Martin for a list of false religions and how they've twisted God's Word to fit their desires. Read *When the World Will Be as One* by Tal Brooke to see how all of these false religions have one thing in common—Satan and "works for salvation."

4 Excerpt from my movie diary.

5 "Half of US Cancer Deaths Due to Bad Habits, Study Finds," aol.com, May 20, 2016, https://www.aol.com/article/2016/05/20/half-of-us-cancer -deaths-due-to-bad-habits-study-finds/21380857/.

6 Up in my bedroom I found this little entry from Valentine's Day 2009 in my devotional.

Devotional 18

1 Find the rest of my song on my website: victoriajackson.com.

Devotional 19

1 William Shakespeare, *Hamlet*, act 1, scene 2. Playing Gertrude, I got to say it in a 1981 performance with John Barrymore III.

2 Victoria Jackson, "It's a Broken World, Baby."

3 Thornton Wilder, *Our Town*.

4 See 1 Corinthians 7.

5 Caroline Leaf.

Devotional 20

1 Christopher Hitchens, The Munk Debate on Religion, Tony Blair vs. Chris Hitchens, Toronto, Canada, 2010.

2 Christopher Hitchens and John Huba, "Topic of Cancer," *Vanity Fair*, August 2010, http://www.vanityfair.com/culture/2010/09/hitchens -201009.

3 TheSasss1, "Christopher Hitchens on Charlie Rose—On His Life and Battling Cancer (August 13, 2010)," YouTube, January 09, 2012, https:// www.youtube.com/watch?v=MtZXmM0uGig.

4 Steve Martin, Goodreads, https://www.goodreads.com/ quotes/71836-it-s-so-hard-to-believe-in-anything-anymore-i-mean.

5 Steve Martin, "Does God Exist?", reprinted at http://www.pbs.org/wgbh /questionofgod/voices/martin.html.

6 Wikipedia contributors, "Steve Martin," Wikipedia, https://en.wikipedia .org/wiki/Steve_Martin.

7 Quoted in Tom Kershaw, "The Religion and Political Views of Steve Martin," *The Hollowverse*, http://hollowverse.com/steve-martin/footnote _3_8002.

8 https://www.lwf.org/daily-treasures/posts/faitha-gift-from-god.

Devotional 21

1 Find the rest of the song on YouTube—a must-see.

Finish Well

1 Nancy Missler, "Faith Is Trusting God," The King's High Way Ministries, 2011, http://www.kingshighway.org/inspiration/articles/sanctification /faith-is-trusting-god/.

2 Find the song on my website: victoriajackson.com.

12/17

VICTORIAJACKSON.COM